MW01706152

A Teenager's Guide to Life

Printed in Canada

ISBN 978-0-9876724-0-7

FIN 05 03 12

Artwork and cover design by Nick White

Library and Archives Canada Cataloguing in Publication

Head Shrinker, D., 1973-

A teenager's guide to life : the secret to living life and being happy / D. Head Shrinker.

ISBN 978-0-9876724-0-7

1. Happiness in adolescence--Popular works. 2. Teenagers-- Conduct of life--Popular works. 3. Adolescent psychology-- Popular works. 4. Self-help techniques for teenagers--Popular works. I. Title.

BF724.3.H35H43 2011 155.5'182 C2011-904024-7

A Teenager's Guide to Life

Where you will find...

The secret to living life

and being happy

Actually, the secret to living isn't that much of a secret. It's quite simple really - inhale... then exhale... then repeat again and again and again and again and... well, I'm sure you get the picture. The secret to being happy, however, is a different story. It is definitely a little more elusive. Unfortunately, if you look around at the people you know (friends, family, the everyday teenager or adult, etc.) it's pretty obvious from its conspicuous absence that it's not common knowledge... which is both unfortunate and surprising since it's not that hard to achieve... once you know what it means to be happy and have instructions on how to get it.

That's what this book is mostly about - an instruction manual for your 'self' and for life in general - so that you can get there - be happy and satisfied with yourself and with life. LEGIT!

Chapter 1

Who the Heck is This Guy?

Welcome to the Jungle

Do you ever wonder "**Why…**"? Why is everything becoming more complicated for you? Why is it that the way you see the world and think about things is changing? Why are there so many questions in your head about life? Why are your friends changing? Why are your friends NOT changing? Why are they acting that way? Why are your parents so…..? Why are they acting that way? Why does anything matter? Why does everything matter? Why did you do that thing that you didn't mean to do? Why is it so hard to feel like you fit in… somewhere… anywhere? Why is it so hard for you to feel comfortable in your own skin? Why do those thoughts pop into your head? Why are your emotions so intense? Why should you spend your time reading this? Why…? Why…? Why…?

If you want to change the rules of life for you and give yourself an unfair advantage over everyone else, then you should read this book. This book is all about understanding ***why***. I can answer all of those questions for you… but only if you really want to know. Only if you want to know why people – people you know, people you care about – **DO** the things that they do. Only if you want to know more about life than your parents do and be able to master the art of "living" and "being happy" in a way that they never did. Only if you want to end up being in control of your life, your happiness, and your future. Only if you want to have a choice in life… a choice most adults have never had and most of your friends will not have (unless they also read this and find out the secret of "living" and "being happy" too).

Now if you are one of the few "good kids" (not much teenage drama in your life, not into sex, drugs and rock n' roll, still thinking that your parents are the most awesome people in the world and thinking how amazingly lucky you are to have them as parents… or whatever…), maybe you are wondering what kind of forbidden knowledge might be in here… maybe you're wondering if you should warn your parents about this book… or check with them first to make sure that it's OK for you to read? By all means, please do! Just keep in mind that they might not give it back to you until they have finished reading it… and maybe giving it to their friends to read… and then rereading it…and then… well, the fact is that you may never get it back. But don't worry if they try to do that. Just go ahead and steal it back (since it is yours) and tell them that there is a version of this book for them too and that they should read theirs rather than yours. (*Their version is a lot more boring and a lot bigger too*).

Now it's possible that, by now (since by 4 paragraphs you've already exceeded the average teenager's attention span by 3 paragraphs), you're wondering if you should continue spending your free time by reading this... or maybe you're wondering if I am some sort of strange, deranged, nut-job... (I mean seriously... what kind of idiot claims to know everything there is to know about life, and how to be happy.... And even if I did, why would I be willing to give this information away for free to anyone who asked?). Does this sound too good to be true? Are you wondering "What's the catch"?

Well, the catch is that... there is no catch. The reason why I have written this and published it and give it away and e-mail it to anyone who wants it is because I am a doctor – a Child and Adolescent Psychiatrist (*a.k.a. a Head Shrinker*) to be exact. And while I do like working with kids and teenagers, I like being on vacation even better. Unfortunately, there are so many unhappy teenagers out there that I'm too busy to go on vacation. So I wrote this book in order to help teenagers figure out how to be happy... so that they can stop wondering if life is worth it... so that they can stop being scared of the future and of life and growing up... so that they can stop making all of those stupid mistakes that they wish they could take back. Basically, I want to change the world – one teenager at a time (*oh yeah... did I mention that I have a little bit of a God Complex?* ☺ *and that I will also require 10% of your life's earnings down the road from now on... you are getting sleepy... sooooooo sleepy.... When I snap my fingers, you will wake up and not remember... ummmm... that uhhh.... thing... that thing that you will forget...* ☺...). I want to give you the chance to be happy that your parents never had. And I also want to not have to work as much and go on vacation a lot more! ☺

Have you ever noticed that most people seem to simply go through life... going through the motions without really enjoying it? It seems like most of the time even 'normal' adults aren't completely satisfied and 'happy' with their lives (i.e. with their jobs, their relationships, their kids, and stuff they have). Granted, they don't seem to be necessarily *unhappy* but the point is that they don't seem to feel **fulfilled** when they think about how their lives have turned out so far. A lot of the time, they don't feel like they are the ones who decided where their lives ended up or even how they got there. In essence, most people wouldn't say that they are **"happy"** and satisfied with life.

I used to be an adult psychiatrist. In my practice, I used to see so much unhappiness and so much confusion about life, and how to live, and how to be happy (_and in a couple of the nurses and other doctors too... *chuckle* - but they weren't my patients_). Now, as an adult psychiatrist, I tried to help them... tried to explain to them how to be happy and in control of their lives... but for the most part, it was too late. They had been thinking about themselves and the world in a particular way for sooooo long that they often could NOT change it. Some of the things that I heard from them over and over and over were things like "I wish someone had told me this stuff back when I was a teenager..." or "Where were you 20 years ago?" or "Why didn't anyone tell me this back when I was a kid? My life would have been sooooooo different..." And so, I stopped treating adults and shifted my focus to treating and helping kids (by helping their parents learn this stuff so that they could teach it to their kids later), and teenagers (by teaching this directly to them).

In my practice, I start by helping teenagers to *understand* the world and the people in it. Then, once they understand that, they start applying that knowledge introspectively and start understanding themselves, their behaviour, and their emotions. After that, they then learn how to control their behaviour and emotions and once they can do that, they suddenly find that their life is much easier, more satisfying, and that they are much more in control of it. In essence, they become happy and satisfied with their lives... and best of all, they stay that way even years later.

Now, if you want to, you can share this with your parents or any adult really. Go ahead and let them read it if you like – they won't disagree with the information that's in this book though they might tell you that they wish that they had had this information when they were a teenager. Or they might steal this book for themselves and not give it back to you. ☺

Chapter 2

Why Are They Doing That?

a.k.a.

What Controls Behaviour?

Why??? … … … … Why Not?!?

I'm going to start by explaining why people (children, teenagers and adults) do the things that they do, say the things that they say, and behave the way they do. In other words, I'm going to tell you what it is that controls ALL human behaviour. Now I'm not talking about which brain structures or neurons do what, I'm talking about the *REASONS…* about what *motivates/makes* us **do stuff.** I'm going to explain why we eat, why we drink, why we talk to people… or not, why we work… or not, why we get dressed in the morning… or not, why we brush our teeth… or not, why we go to school… or not, why we watch TV… or not, why we listen to music… or not, why we dance… or not, why we play… or not, why we love… or not, why we have sex… or not, why we pretend… or not, why we fantasize… or not, why we imagine… or not, why we think… or not … and… why we want to… no… ***need to*** know ***why***.

If you think about human behaviour and all of the things that people do and are capable of doing, you're probably going to be surprised when I tell you that there are really only **two** things that control our behaviour. Are you ready?

"There are really only **two** things that control our behaviour".

Was I right? Are you surprised? Wanna know more? Then read on.

(*Actually … it's really about* 2.584592 *parts… but I'm rounding. My goal in writing this book is to help eventually build a generation of 3s… or 1s depending on how you look at it. … just give me a minute and I'll explain what that means… then you'll understand*).

(*Hmmm… I just had a thought [I do that every now and then]… I think that would make an awesome good T-shirt! I should totally get a bunch of Ts made up that say* "Generation 3… or 1 … depending on how you look at it" *on the back, but in a much cooler font of course… like maybe the 'Halo' font…what do you think?*

Generation 3
… or 1 …
depending on how you look at it

And then, just for fun, make some other Ts that say “Generation 2.584592” *that you can give to your parents - you know - for like Christmas or their birthday or something… *chuckle*. And the best part is that they'll have no clue.* .

OK… that was kind of random… Anyways, back to what I was explaining… (but I am totally going to do that… thanks for the idea.)(e-mail me[1] *if you want me to send you one*).

OK. So then… where was I……. RIGHT! The two things in our brains that make us act. These two parts of our brain are biologically based *drives* or *needs* – like the *need* to eat, the *need* to drink, the *need* to stay warm and maintain our body temperature. These two drives are the Harm-Avoidance Drive and the Pleasure-Seeking Drive.

These two drives are essentially *information processing modules* that each have a ***Prime Directive***; a *reason* for their existence… the one thing that they have to do… or in other words, their *goal in life*. The Prime Directive for the Harm Avoidance Drive is… to ***Avoid Harm***[2] while the Prime Directive for the Pleasure Seeking Drive is … can you guess? That's right… *it's to sing badly out of key during Karaoke night!!! … no… wait…. Sorry… I was thinking about a different part of the brain… ignore what I just said…* It's to ***Go Get Good Stuff*** [*sorry about all of the technical jargon…*].

Now *'Good Stuff'* is not necessarily what you might think it is…

“?!?”

---

[1] Generation3or1@rogers.com

[2] In other words, stay away from *'Bad Stuff'* [*this is the scientific term*]. For all the math-brained people reading this, let me put it a different way: Harm = *'Bad Stuff'*… I know… this is getting complicated… but bear with me.

... OK, yeah... that is some of the stuff that would be considered *Good Stuff*...

"?"

... yep, that too...

"?"

...and yes... dead on!

"?"

... ... ummmmmmm?!?.... OK?!?.... nnnnoooo... ... ... at least not for normal people... (*Who let him in here?*). *'Good Stuff'* includes all of those things (except for what he said... that's just wrong) but it also includes other things too like winning at a game, being around people, food, water, PS3, music, cigarettes, marijuana, partying, physical contact, and pretty much anything that you would consider *'sick'* (not the doctor 'sick'... or that guy's either!).

The way that these two parts of our brain work are similar – they are both constantly processing the world around us, scanning and analyzing everything that we experience through our 5 senses (everything that we see, hear, smell, taste and touch/feel) comparing what's out there in the world with what's on their respective lists of *Good Stuff* and *Bad Stuff*. Then, as they are filtering through all of this information, if they run across something that matches up with something on their lists (i.e. something 'good' or something 'bad'), they will activate and start directing and controlling what we do, so that they can fulfill their Prime Directive.

Remember when I said that there were only *two* things that controlled us? Well, I sort-of fudged the truth a little (i.e. lied)... but not really... because, you see, in kids, it **is** true, it's only those two drives that control them. And in teenagers & adults, it's still primarily those two drives that control us. **BUT** in adults and teenagers, along with the two drives, there is a third,

critically important part of the brain that comes into play in controlling behaviour.

This third part of the brain only starts to develop around the time that we hit puberty. It isn't there in kids (just like body hair in certain areas... ). This third part of the brain is the ***Logic and Reason Center***. This is the '*thinking*' part of the brain. This part of the brain also has a Prime Directive, which is essentially ***'Don't be Stupid!'***. Most people refer to this part of the brain as "Common Sense". Scientists and Doctors call it by its scientific name which is "The '*No Duh!!!*' Centre".

A useful way to think about these two drives is to think of them as two tiny people that are living in our heads (since birth), giving us orders and telling us what to do (just like parents did when we were kids). How loud they are when they tell us to do something represents how strong or powerful that drive is. The louder they are, the stronger the drive and the stronger the drive, the less control *we* will have. Now because we know these two little people in our heads well (since they have been there since the day we were born), we trust them completely! We don't question them and what they are telling us to do and so, automatically, we will go and do what they are telling us to do. Logic and Reason would be like a third little guy that moves in to your head around puberty and who has been given a mission by Mother Nature... to take over from the other two.

The Logic and Reason centre of the brain is like a sleeper-agent who gets activated when you hit puberty. Once he's activated, he is supposed to take over and be the boss of us... the guy in charge! Funny thing is though... he's not. He's like the smart, 98 pound weakling while the other two are like the massive, 250 pound bullies. When he first gets activated/moves in, whenever he tries to take control of what we do, he always loses because he simply isn't strong enough to take them on. **BUT**, as time goes on, the more he trains and tries to go against them (the two drives), the stronger he becomes. Unfortunately, for most people in the world, when he was first activated he never trained long enough or tried hard enough to become really strong. In most people, when he first tried to take over and couldn't, he often stopped trying so hard and gave up. He would only try half-heartedly when he was in his *prime* (that's where you are right now), when he would be able to get stronger if the effort was there. As a result, for most people, once they are adults and that part of the brain is finished growing, he ends up being roughly 58.4592% as strong as the other two. (*Do the T-shirts make sense now?* ☺)

An analogy that might help to clarify the relationships between these three parts of the brain is to think of a 'human' as being equivalent to a 'village'[3]. This village needs to continue to exist/survive and so they pick a member of the village to be the **Lookout** (LOOKOUT = HARM AVOIDANCE DRIVE OR 'BOB') and someone else to be the **Seeker** (SEEKER = PLEASURE SEEKING DRIVE OR 'JIM'). The **Lookout** is the person who is responsible for standing guard and watching for incoming danger. His job is to notice and recognize dangers and then to tell the rest of the village what to do in order to avoid the danger. The **Seeker** is the person who is responsible for going out and finding food and shelter and other villages full of hotties.[4]

Anyways… it's the Seeker's job to find these things and then go and tell the villagers what to do and where to go to get the food and shelter and potties… I mean hotties. The Logic and Reason Center would be the equivalent of the **Village Chief** – the one who is supposed to have the final say in what the village does (CHIEF = LOGIC AND REASON CENTER OR '*YOU*'). Unfortunately, in this village, the Chief is a baby and so the village will have to wait until he grows up and matures before he will be able to take over and start directing the village's activities. In the interim, the village has to rely on the **Lookout** and on the **Seeker** to take care of them and make sure it survives until the **Chief** grows up.

The following three chapters will look at each of these three parts of the brain in more detail to help you gain an in-depth understanding of them. Understanding how the two drives work is the most important thing because they are so powerful and control so much of what everybody does in life. Everything else that I have to say after explaining them to you assumes that you 'got it' and that you know them really, really well… that

---

3 For all the Math-brained people reading this, think of it this way: HUMAN = VILLAGE

4 *OMG… LMAO… my spell checker just tried to change that last sentence for me… from 'hotties' to 'potties'…* RFLOL

you understand them and how they work and what makes them tick. This is especially true when I get to the part of this book that explains how *YOU* can manipulate them, mess with them and eventually turn the tables on them and control them. If you don't 'get it' after reading through the next three chapters, then put the book down and come back to it later and read it again. It's best if you read the next three chapters when you are calm, rested and fed. If you are tired, cranky, emotional, or hungry, you won't be able to process the information as well and it will be harder to 'get it'. If you decide that you don't really care enough to try to understand it well, then you don't get it... and you'll qualify for a "Generation 2.584592" T-shirt in a few years.

As you read through each chapter, you will notice that I go back and forth between referring to the drives as "he" and as "it".

THAT'S BECAUSE WE HAVE A SPLIT PERSONALITY.

I do not!

YES WE DO!

Liar! ...

NO, YOU ARE!

Shut up!!!

NO YOU SHUT UP!!!

... ...

Sorry about that. Just ignore him.

As I was saying, I switch back and forth between **'he'** and **'it'** because it is important to remember a couple of things about these drives. I use **'he'** to emphasize the fact that even though these two drives are biologically part of our brain and our body, they are not under our control. ***We*** don't decide what ***they*** do (it's actually the other way around most of the time...). ***They*** are not *us* and do not represent *'US'* – *Who* **we** are. What ***they*** tell us (i.e. what they think/say) is **not the same** as what ***we*** think.

It is exactly like having 2 other people controlling us like we are just puppets!

I also use the term '**it**' to emphasize the fact that these two drives are ***just*** a couple of ***machines*** (information processing modules – like a computer). They have a very strict set of rules (their Prime Directives) that they have to follow no matter what. They simply react to information without taking into account (*thinking about*) ***context*** (the circumstances). They are as dumb as stumps. Remembering these two facts is critical and is going to be especially important when I explain why you should fight them to gain control and how to do it so that you win.

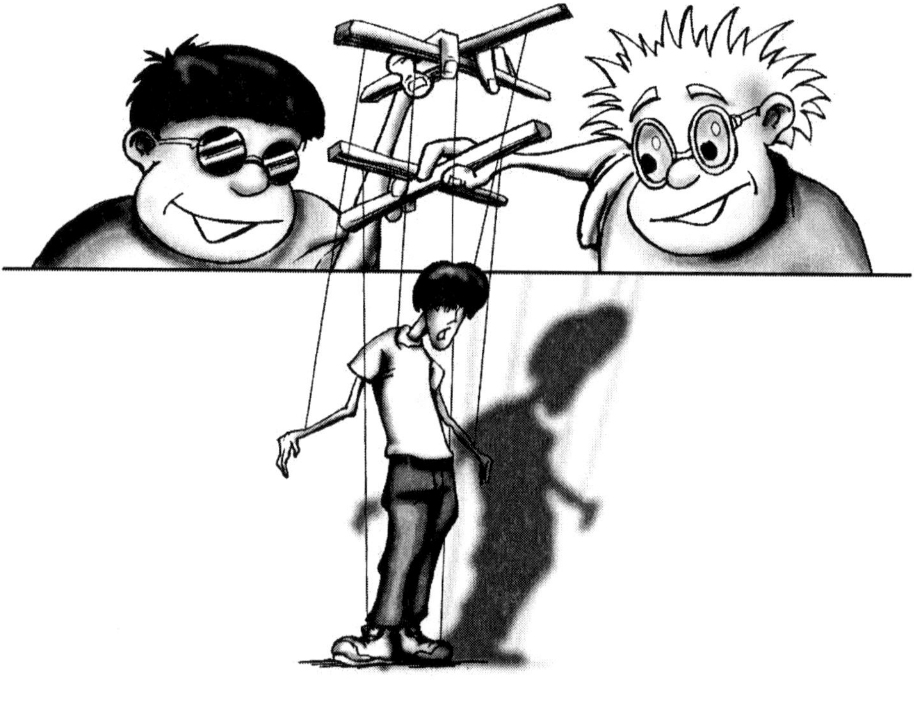

Chapter 3

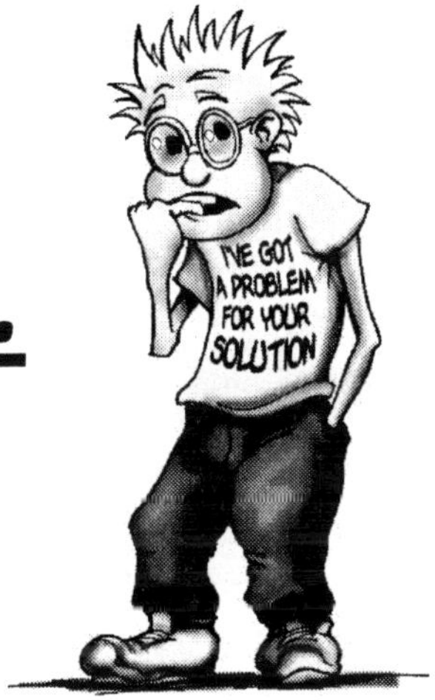

Introducing... BOB!!!

a.k.a.

The Harm Avoidance Drive

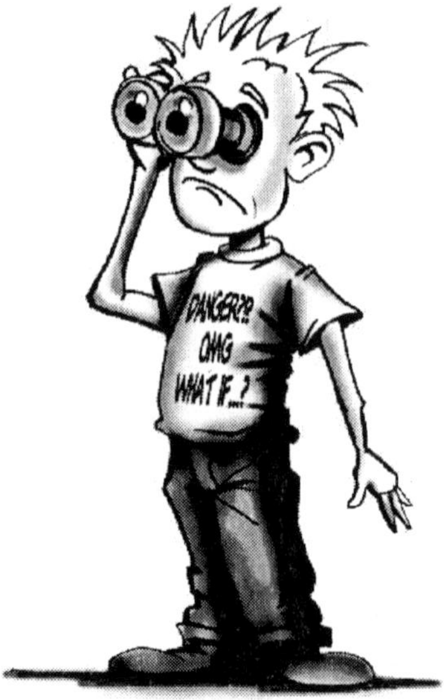

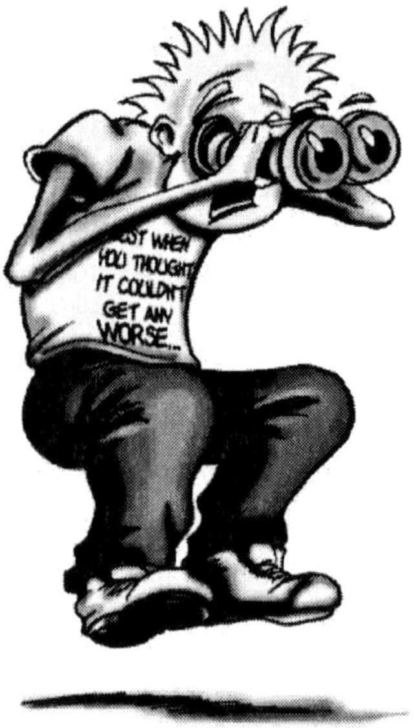

The Harm Avoidance Drive a.k.a "Bob"

The Harm Avoidance Drive – I call him "Bob" – *(b/c it's much faster to type 'Bob' than 'The Harm Avoidance Drive')*[5] is the part of our brain that is designed to function as a defence system. It's there so that it can protect us from danger. Bob's Prime Directive is ***"Avoid Bad Stuff"***. In order to do this, he spends every minute of every day constantly monitoring and tracking *everything* around us – everything that we see, hear, taste, smell, touch/feel/sense (in other words, **everything** that we experience in our lives) looking out for *Bad Stuff*. When Bob sees *Bad Stuff*, he sends us an IM[6] telling us what to do to take evasive action – to make sure that we avoid that bad/dangerous thing.

---

[5] ***[Editor's Note: We think this is stupid and confusing!!!].***
[Author's Note: We think that the editors are stupid and confusing!!!].

[6] *IM = Instant Message - as if I really have to explain what an IM is... sheeesh... but my editor thinks that you guys won't have a clue what* ***'all the weird acronyms'*** *mean... I assured him that you would understand what IM, LOL, LMAO, ROTFLMAO, OMG and stuff like that meant... [that's what an acronym is btw.] so I'm humouring him and spelling it out - in case your parents read this I guess...*

Now, as I was saying earlier, the term *Bad stuff* is a complex scientific term that is used to describe an extremely complicated part of our brain. I'm going to try to explain it in a little bit more detail for you, while keeping it simple enough to understand[7]. OK. So. When I use the term *Bad Stuff*, I am referring to a *big list of **bad things** in our brain* (it's a type of 'memory' in our brain). Some of the things on this list were there the minute we were born (*Yes, you can be born knowing that celery is bad, disgusting and overall as useless a vegetable as any that has ever walked the earth... not that celery walks or anything.. but you know what I mean...right?)*

YOU'RE AN IDIOT... WALKING CELERY???? WHAT CRACK ARE YOU SMOKING!

I said SHUT UP!

WHATEVER CELERY BOY...

GO AWAY!!! No-one asked for your opinion!

SO ?!? YOUR POINT IS???? ...

As I was saying... (... *that guy is such a pain in my... *sigh*)*... some of the things are on that list because we were born with them on it while the rest of the things on that list are there because they got added to the list as a result of life. Another way to think about it is that some of the stuff on this list was there *before* we were born and the rest got added to it *after* we were born. :-D *(And to think that I figured that out all by myself! Me much very smart eh!?![8]).*

Oh yeah, I forgot to mention that the stuff that gets added to this list *after* we are born is the *Bad Stuff* that we personally experience in our lives. This includes all of that *Bad Stuff* that we didn't know was bad until we

---

[7] *But please keep in mind that I am a doctor - I went to doctor school for a long time to learn a bunch of other stuff that has nothing to do with any of this... *chuckle* ... you know, after you read and understand this, you will likely know more about what controls behaviour than most regular doctors do!*

[8] *I'm Canadian in case any non-Canadians are wondering about the 'eh' thing... Weird eh?*

experienced it in some fashion. That could mean that it happened to us and we experienced all the unpleasantness first hand [**the best way to get put on '*The List*'**] *(think celery...)*, or it could mean that we saw it happen to someone else [*a pretty good way to get put on 'The List'*] or it could mean that we heard or read about it happening to someone else, somewhere else [maybe it gets on *'The List'*... or maybe not...]. (*This is usually how Broccoli and Brussels Sprouts end up on the list*).

How many times Bob messages or texts us depends on how BIG and **BAD** he thinks the *Bad Stuff* is and how far away it is (time or distance). The bigger + the badder + the closer = the more he messages and texts us and the bigger and bigger his messages get and the louder he is when he finally calls us on his cell phone to yell at us – if we weren't responding to his texts.

To give you an example of what the Bob looks like in action, let's pretend that your Bob has spiders on its list and has it ranked as pretty freakingly not good. Maybe spiders are on his list because he was born with it on there or maybe because it was added after you were born (i.e. when you were kid, you were attacked by a horde of tarantulas

...OH PLEASE, IT WAS ONE LOUSY TARANTULA...

and barely escaped with your life; or maybe one day when you were a kid, your dad saw a spider and **HE** screamed like a terrified little girl and ran away in a panic to hide in the bedroom

HE'S TALKING ABOUT HOW HE REACTED IN FRONT OF HIS DAUGHTER... LMAO...

and that was when you realized that this horrible, monstrous beast was a HUGE, BAD, VERY, VERY, **VERY** DANGEROUS THING... since it was so deadly that it terrified even your father![9] ... or maybe there is absolutely no ***reason*** for it being on that list – Bob just decided to mess with you so he put it on that list just for kicks... a practical joke gone bad).

---

[9] And also because everything we know about life, we learned from our parents – I'll explain more about that in a later chapter.

Either way, at the end of the day, it doesn't really matter why it's on the list. Just imagine that it is... and it's highlighted as being very, very BAAAAADDDDDD... and it's on the list in six different places. Or another way of saying this is "Imagine that you have *Arachnophobia.*[10]". Now because you have Arachnophobia, Bob is **ALWAYS** watching out for spiders.

Now, close your eyes *(not yet... it makes it really hard to read if you do! - wait until I finish telling you what to picture in your head!)* and imagine yourself doing something – anything at all – and then imagine that a ***huge, hairy spider*** suddenly drops down from the ceiling, twirling on its web, right in front of your nose. *(OK, now close your eyes and imagine that!)*. How would you react? What do you think you would do?

HE FREAKS OUT AND SCREAMS LIKE A LITTLE GIRL!!! ROTFLMAO!!!

I do not!!! ... any more...

YOU USED TO!

That was a long time ago! ... Whatever... (I really hate that guy!!! He's a total loser!)

Anyways, if this happened to you, and you had Arachnophobia, you would be "***freaking out***"[11]! Now hit Pause on that mental picture that's in your head and let's take a closer look at what's happening.

What you are doing right at that moment (your behavioural response to the spider – a.k.a 'Freaking out'), has one goal and one goal only – to take evasive action... to do whatever it takes to get away from that spider... *because* Bob's yelling at you on his phone saying "OMG OMG OMG GET AWAY!!! RUN!!!! GET HELP!!!!!" ... *because* Bob's list of *Bad Stuff* has

[10] *It's a big doctory Latin word that, if you translate it in Google Translator back to English, would be "spider fear". Did you know it takes 13 years of doctor school to be able to make that "formal" diagnosis? lol*

[11] *"Freaking out" = jumping backwards, waving your hands frantically (doggie-paddle-like) in front of your face, trying to get away... and yes... maybe sometimes..., screaming like a girl.*

'spiders' on it and spiders are highlighted as being dangerous... ***deadly***... *It's-going-to-kill-you* bad!!! *Muwhhaahhhahha. *insert evil laugh here*.*

Note: Exam question coming up! It's very important to understand this next paragraph so pay attention!

Now, **right at that point in time** when you are screaming, jumping back, running away or otherwise "freaking out", **things that are normally under *YOUR* voluntary control** – like the movement of *your* muscles, *your* voice, *your* body – these things **stopped being under your control!** At no point in time did *you* ***decide*** to 'freak out' like that. You just did – automatically, almost instantaneously, as soon as Bob saw it. In fact, not only did you not *choose* to freak out, but **EVEN IF YOU DID NOT WANT TO...** (even if ***you*** were determined that this time, you would not jump back and scream like a girl but instead, *this time*, you would just calmly look at the spider and maybe even let it land on your nose... or even just your hand...) **YOU WOULD NOT BE ABLE TO MAKE YOURSELF NOT FREAK-OUT!!!** You would not be *able to ignore* the orders that Bob yelled at you when he called your cell in a panic. Simply put, as far as your brain is concerned, **you *are not allowed* to ignore him**... it's for your own good!

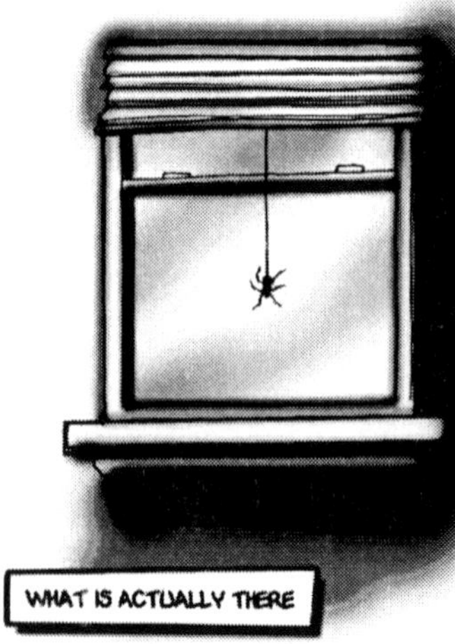

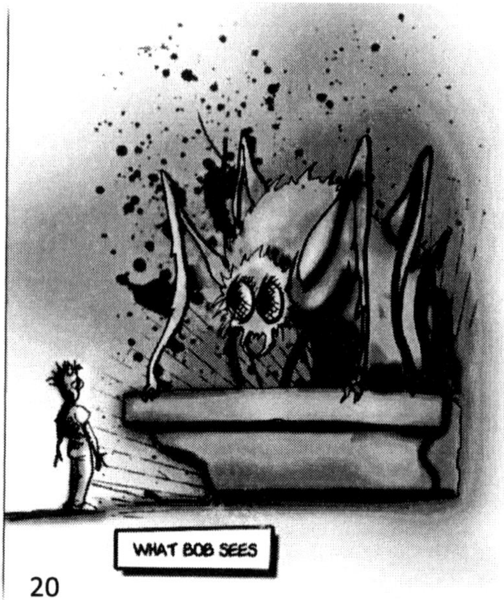

WHETHER OR NOT IT IS ACTUALLY DANGEROUS, FOR REALLY-FOR-REAL, DOES NOT MATTER ONE BIT! IF IT IS ON BOB'S LIST AND THE LIST SAYS IT'S "DEADLY DANGEROUS", THEN AS FAR AS BOB'S CONCERNED, IT IS DEADLY AND HE'S GOING TO REACT LIKE YOUR BODY'S CONTINUED EXISTENCE (LIFE) LITERALLY DEPENDS ON HIM MAKING YOU DO WHATEVER HE TELLS YOU TO DO.

OK. Now, I want to fill you in on Bob – how he works, why he insists on you calling him 'Robert', why he's always mooching money off you, why he thinks that you are just kidding when you tell him to go away, about the time he got drunk at the X-mas party and ended up falling over into the punch bowl, why you can't get him to shut up, why he acts and thinks like a two year old... ... ... *(oh wait... sorry... wrong Bob. I was thinking of a surgeon I know. Sorry about that)*. Hmmm... well, actually, the last two do fit the Harm-Avoidance Drive... especially the last one. Bob (the Harm-Avoidance Drive, not the surgeon) is as dumb as a stump![12] He is a moron's moron. Ask him ***why*** he thinks that doing something is a good idea and his answer is most likely to be "Cuz I said so..." or "Huh?... What?... I don't get it..." or "   ". Oh yeah... and he also can't count!

Things Bob can do:

1) *Manage/maintain and update the list of "Bad Stuff".*

   The *Bad Stuff* list is basically a collection of little 'pictures' or 'snapshots' of all of the sensory information associated with bad things – what you were seeing/hearing/tasting/feeling/sensing at the time that the bad thing happened (which sometimes has absolutely nothing at all to do with the actual bad thing) - based on ***your experience*** of those bad things. Whenever you experience something that you do not like (a.k.a. 'Bad') in your life, Bob takes a quick snapshot of everything that you are seeing,

[12] *Mind you, so is the other Bob... but that's got nothing to do with this Bob...*

hearing, smelling, touching or tasting (sensory information) when the bad thing happened and adds it to the list. Depending on what has happened in your life and how keen Bob is at doing his job, his list of *Bad Stuff* can be very **BIG** or very small.

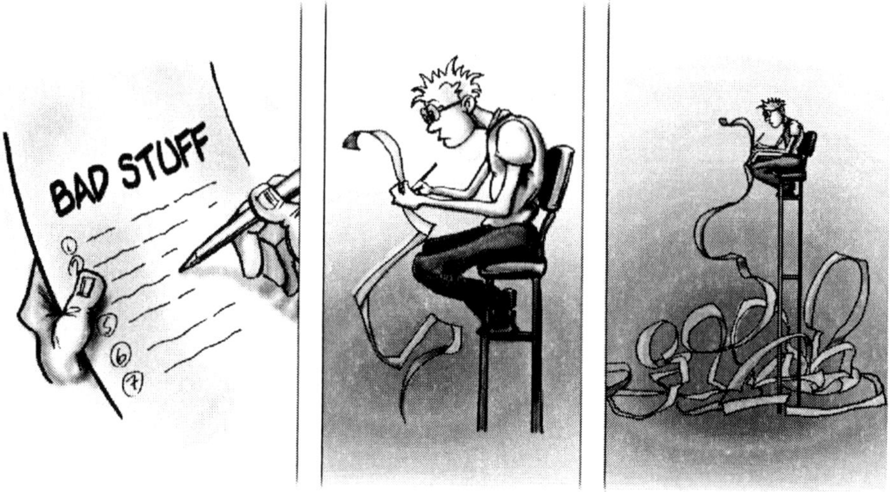

2) *Review and tell you all about the stuff that's on his list of "Bad Stuff".*
He can send you a message containing that information or call you on his cell to tell you all about it over the phone. Oh yeah, he also only knows one number – yours! And he knows how to hit redial... and speed dial... over and over and over if need be; after all, you're the only one he ever calls! (*Poor Bob*)...

3) *Make you to listen to him, believe him and do what he says.*
This is because Bob's actually kinda scary to talk to! When he calls, he is always yelling, freaking out, catastrophizing[13], panicking and telling you that you are going to die if you don't listen to him and do what he says. And most of the time, you'll listen to him very quickly just to make him shut up and leave you alone.

[13] Making mountains out of molehills and molehills out of nothing.

Things Bob cannot do:

1) Count
2) Think
3) Understand "time"
4) Understand anything
5) Think
6) Analyze information (above and beyond just matching up the stuff out there with the stuff on his list of *Bad Stuff*)
7) Think
8) **NOT** be an idiot

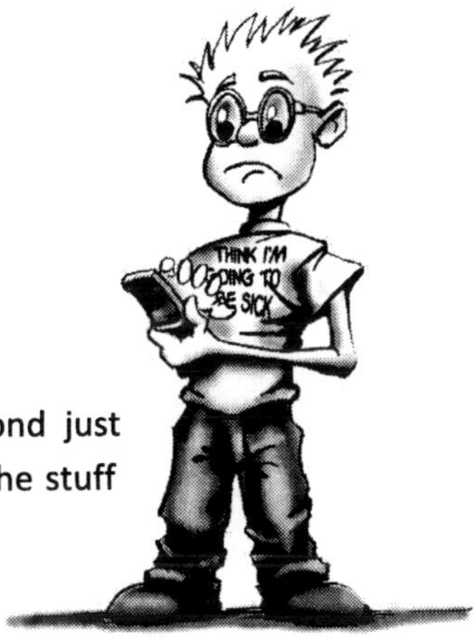

Unfortunately, even though Bob's an idiot, he's kinda like your childhood BFF[14]; because you've known him your whole life, you trust him COMPLETELY.[15] You believe that he is **always** right about what he's telling you is dangerous and what he's telling you to do about it. The problem for you is that sometimes (a lot of times actually), he really-for-real ***isn't right*** and in fact, is often really-for-real dead wrong when he is talking about either the stuff on his list *actually* being bad!!! And to make matters worse, even when he happens to be right about something on the list and it is really-for-real 'bad', the stuff he tells you to do to avoid it will often make no sense at all and often don't work to avoid the danger... and can even seriously mess up your life and make it worse when you do what he says to do.

Did I mention yet that animals have Harm Avoidance Drives too? And that their Bobs works just like our Bobs do... and are just as *smart* too! Think about that!!! *YOUR* Bob's smarts = *BAMBI'S* Bob's smarts. Let me spell it out for you... ... When Bambi's Bob sees something that matches something on his list, he calls Bambi on his little Bambi cell phone and might say stuff like "DON'T MOVE!!!" or "FREEZE!!!". Now this is a fine strategy if what Bob saw was a predator like a wolf (they notice movement

---

[14] *BFF = Best Friend Forever .... Duh...*

[15] Even though it's really not much fun when he calls you and, in fact, you hate hearing from him and really don't "like" him.

really well) but not such a great idea If Bambi is crossing a highway at night.[16] In that situation, freezing and stopping in the middle of the road is not really the best way to avoid bad stuff... and in fact, almost guarantees something really-for-real bad happening (I think it's safe to assume that Bambi becoming road-kill would be a bad thing for Bambi). Same thing with an ostrich that buries it's head in the sand when it senses danger... because if you can't see it, then it's not there and it's no longer dangerous... right??? Yeah, right!

Did I also mention yet that our Harm-Avoidance Drive (Bob) still works much the same as animals' do? Yeah I did! (*Weren't you paying attention?*). Well, it's still true! (*It has to be... I said it twice now!*) Even though we consider ourselves to be a highly evolved species...

"... ?"

Yes, I mean "humans"... (*Dear god, there's always one in every group!*). Unfortunately, even in humans, Bob still hasn't developed much in the way of intelligence. The most common order/instruction that he yells at us is "FREEZE!!!" and "DON'T!" – don't go there, don't do that, don't eat that, don't say that, don't act that way, don't move.... Most of the time, Bob freezes us, paralyzes us and ***stops us*** from doing stuff.

"?"

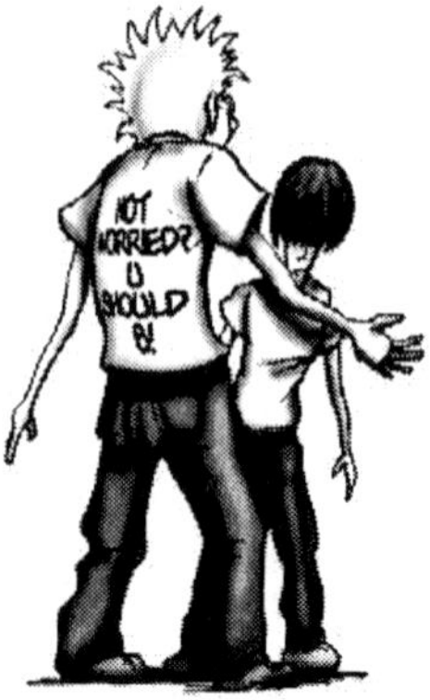

Yes, just like he does with Bambi.

Afraid of getting the answer wrong on a test? Bob's solution: don't write anything down... then it can't be wrong... *right*?

Afraid of asking someone out and having them say no... and being alone (i.e. not having a girl/boyfriend)? Bob's solution: don't ask them...then they won't

[16] Bob: *Lookit dat dere big pair of eyes* [**headlights**] *on dat dere biggum predator* [**Mack Truck**]. *I Better call Bambi and warn him!* "BAMBI.... DON'T MOVE or else he'll see you and eat you!"

say no... and you won't be alone... *right*??
Afraid of people not liking you? Bob's solution: don't go hang out with people, don't leave your room... then people will like you... *right*???

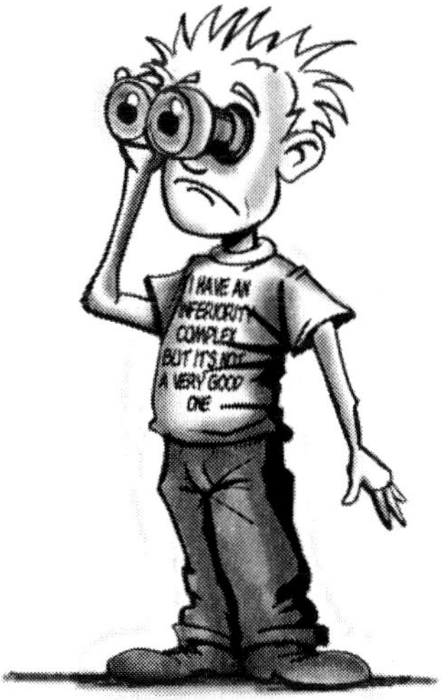

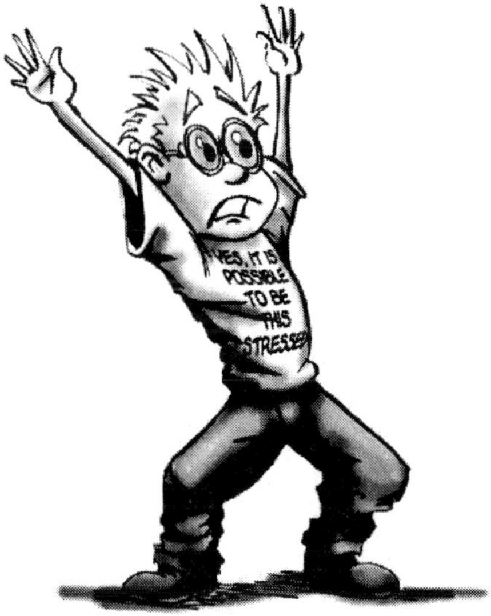

Other important things to know about Bob:

1) He moves in the day we are born and will be there until the day we die. He works 24/7/365.
2) The battery on Bob's cell phone sucks which means that even though he can call us and yell at us, he can only actually talk to us for a limited time. His battery runs out after about 45 minutes... ish... then he has to recharge it for another 10-15 minutes before being able to call us again.
3) His work ethic – how busy he is and how good he is at doing his job of noticing *Bad Stuff*, adding information on that *Bad Stuff* to his list and texting/calling you – depends mainly on your parents. You see, 'Bob' (our Harm-Avoidance Drives) is mostly something that you inherit. The Harm-Avoidance Drive exists in a very specific, physical chunk of gooey stuff in our heads and fortunately/unfortunately, what our bodies are like – what we look like, the colour of our hair, the colour of our eyes, how tall

we are, and, yes, what our Bob's chunk of goo is like – depends mostly on what our parents' bodies/brains are like.[17]

[17] *In other words, it's something you inherited from them. Just like diarrhea … it runs in the jeans!*

Chapter 4

Introducing…
JIM!!!

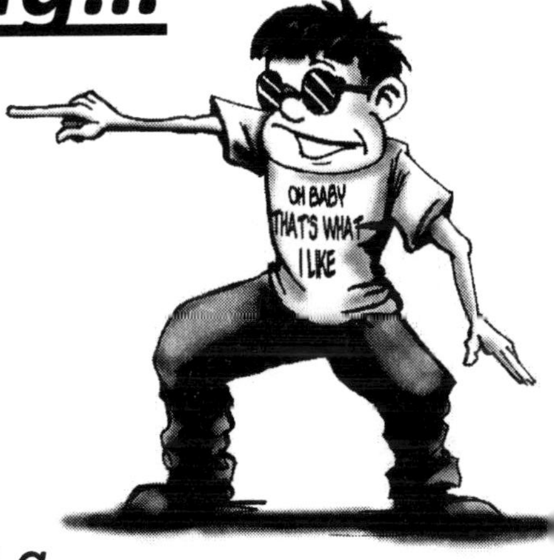

a.k.a.

The Pleasure Seeking Drive

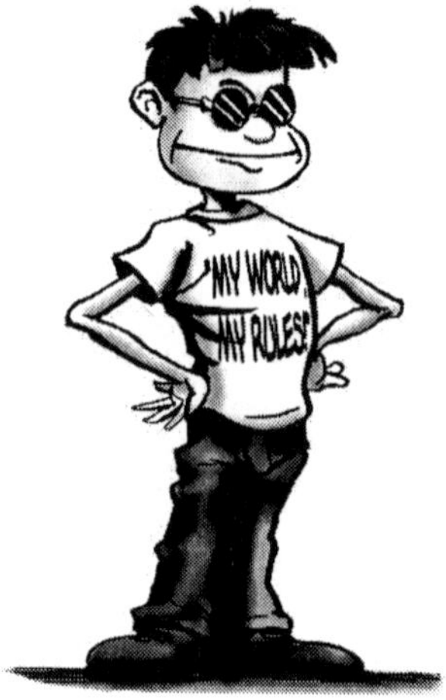

The Pleasure Seeking Drive (a.k.a. "Jim")

The Pleasure Seeking Drive, who I call "Jim",[18] is the other one you need to know about. (Remember? We're talking about the *two* drives that control us... still with me right?). Jim's Prime Directive (his job) is to **Go get *Good Stuff***. *(My editor also thinks I have to repeat what kinds of things = "Good Stuff" in case you didn't read it two chapters ago. I told him this was a book for teenagers, not 2 year olds...) ... ... (page 7 paragraph 1 JIC[19])...*

So then, *Good Stuff* is yet another complex scientific term that is used to describe another extremely complicated system in our brain (just like *Bad Stuff* was). When I use the term *Good Stuff*, I am referring to a big list of GOOD THINGS in our brain. *(You've probably noticed that I basically cut and pasted this sentence from the last chapter where I explained what Bad Stuff was - that's cuz the way these two lists work is basically the same - stuff on it before birth, stuff on it after birth, used as a reference for comparison for Jim when he is trying to match up the stuff he sees on the screen in our brains to the list of*

---

18 **[Editor's Note: We still think this is stupid and confusing!!!]**
[Author's note: And we still think that the editor is stupid and confusing... and has really, really bad B.O. too!]
[Editor's Note: What's B.O. stand for?]
[Author's note: 😁]

19 *JIC = Just In Case... JIC you didn't know that...*

Good Stuff so he can tell what kind of stuff out there is Good Stuff... blah blah blah...). Anyways...

All the stuff on the list of *Good Stuff* has one thing in common: everything that is on that list makes our brain go " WHEEEEEEEEEE!!!!!! ". Which basically means that there is Dopamine being released in our brain. Dopamine is our brain's *universal Good Stuff indicator.*[20] To put it in simple terms, Dopamine in brain = "liking"[21] = Jim taking a snapshot of all sensory input when Dopamine levels went up and pasting all that information into his list of *Good Stuff*. If you "like" *(not lick... LOL)* something, anything, that means that it is on that list of *Good Stuff*. Can you guess what it means if you "don't like" something... which list it's on?

"?"

What???.... NO!... Who... You again???... How did you get back in here?....

... **sigh*... OMG... some people....*

Just like Bob, when Jim sees something on his screen that matches up with something on his list of *Good Stuff*, he does the same thing as Bob does and messages/texts you to let you know he found something relevant to his job and then tells you what you have to do to go and get it. Jim is like our other BFF that we trust completely (except that we really "like" it when Jim does his job) and so we go ahead and do what he tells us to do. It's because of Jim that we can't stop at just one chip... one cookie... one bite of that yummy cake.

Jim is the reason why we get 'addicted' to things. When we say that someone is 'addicted' to something, that means two things: 1) it means that Jim is telling them that (a.k.a. "they feel like") the thing that they are 'addicted' to is **SOOOOOOOOOOOOO** important to them that they **have to have/do it!** And even if they decide to[22] try to stop having/doing whatever

---

[20] Once again for the math-brained people: IF <u>*insert name of thing here*</u> = Dopamine in brain, **THEN** <u>*insert name of thing here*</u> = *Good Stuff.*

[21] ... *my spell checker didn't catch my last typo... "liking" was in there as "<u>licking</u>"... ... I can just imagine how confusing that would have been... lol.*

[22] Once the Logic and Reason Center matures

it is, they can't. In other words, **Jim wins no matter what.** The second criterion used to define the term addicted is that the thing that Jim is telling them to do is bad for them and causes problems for them in their lives. In other words, it makes no sense at all for them to have/do that thing! Unfortunately, when Jim (the Pleasure-Seeking Drive) gets to the point of actually *calling* us, and talking to us, it's soooooooo hard not to listen to him. He is **SOOOOOOO** convincing when he wants to be... he can basically talk us into doing just about anything... and have us believing that it was our idea in the first place.

When Jim (the Pleasure-Seeking Drive) first starts working (in other words, when we are born), the only stuff that is on his list of *Good Stuff* is stuff that ***really is critical for our survival*** as an individual and as a species (stuff like food, water, warmth, physical contact, sex, grouping up [herding – like sheep or dogs or horses....], and 'winning' [moving up in the 'pecking order' a.k.a. improving your social 'standing' a.k.a. getting closer to being the 'Boss Dog' or 'Head honcho' or 'Leader'). Then, as we go through life, if we experience something good (which causes dopamine to be released in our brains), it gets added to the list. In our lives, as long as Jim gets stuff that matches up with stuff on his list of *Good Stuff*, everything's good! *(That wasn't confusing at all... was it?)*

Now, generally speaking, Jim does a good job for the first couple of years of our lives... but there is a problem brewing because of how he identifies *Good Stuff*. You see, every time that we *experience* something that triggers or causes the release of Dopamine in our brain[23], Jim quickly takes a snapshot (picture) of all of the sensory information (what we are seeing, hearing, touching, smelling or tasting) that is associated with this flood of Dopamine in our brains and adds that information to his list. **Whether or not that stuff really *is* important for our survival or not makes no**

[23] Like the first time you inhale a cigarette or try a hit of Cocaine or Ecstasy – because those chemical compounds automatically force Dopamine to be released in our brain thus *tricking our brain* into thinking that that thing is something that it's not... just like artificial sweetener isn't really sugar! The bigger the flood of Dopamine in our brain = the more 'addictive' something is. Oh, btw – how much dopamine is release by certain chemicals is very strongly determined by genetics... which is why addiction problems often run in families. For some people, trying something ***once*** is all it takes for Jim to **LOVE** it and need it more than anything else in the world!!!

difference. This is how stuff like TV, video games, Messengerish-like online chatting things[24], gambling, cigarettes, weed (pot, marijuana, ganja, grass... whatever you know it as), Cocaine, E, other recreational drugs, fetishes and a bunch of other ridiculously useless stuff gets onto that list. And then, because it's on his list, Jim treats it like it is *just as important to our survival as food and water and warmth* – even though in reality, it has absolutely nothing at all to do with our survival... and in some cases (i.e. smoking cigarettes or doing drugs), will do the exact opposite and hurry us along to an early death!

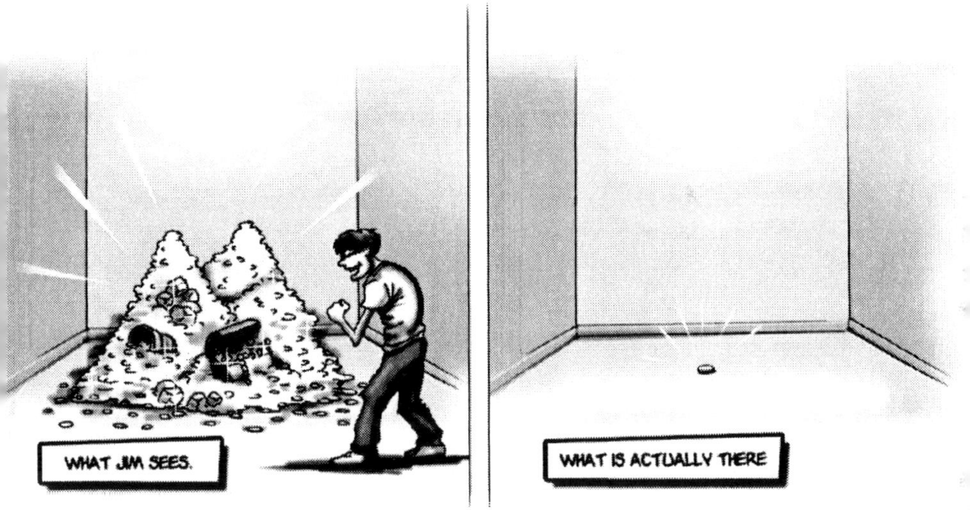

Now, here's the scoop on Jim. He's a lot like Bob – there from day one, with a *List* that can be big or small, and a genetically inherited work ethic. He does his job the same way that Bob does (matching up information out there with stuff on his list and adding info to the list as needed). Oh yeah... Jim's also an idiot too. He's just as dumb as Bob is; he's also a moron's moron[25].

---

[24] *Apparently, "Mr. Legal Department" says I can't use a "Trademarked and Copyrighted" name without permission... yeah... OK... Like I'm sure Bill Gates is going to care if I mention one of his products here...*

[25] *Wow... who knew that editing could be so funny... it's hilarious what the spell-checker misses sometimes. That last sentence was in the original draft as* "a Mormon's moron" *lol].*

Things Jim can do:

1) All the same stuff as Bob (*again, I don't think I need to cut and paste it from the last chapter to here word for word... do I? Go back and look if you need to...*).
2) Always make you to listen to him, believe him and do what he says – same as Bob. However, while Bob is scary and frightens you into doing stuff, Jim is smooth. First, he tries sweet-talking you into it or tells you it was your idea in the first place. Then, if need be, he gets you fired up and angry. He convinces you that it's your *right* to have that *thing...* and that you desperately need to listen to him and go get **it** (whatever it is on his list of *Good Stuff* that he wants you to go and get) if you want to survive... if you want to be King!

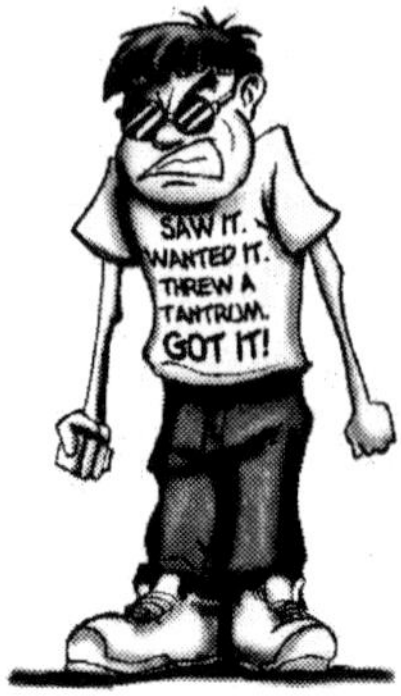

Things Jim cannot do:

1) All the same stuff as Bob (*again, I don't think I need to cut and paste it from the last chapter to here word for word... do I? Go back and look if you need to...*). (GUESS WHAT HE JUST DID... 😒) ... *I did not... well.. ok... maybe I did...*

BUT the *way* Jim does his job is a little bit different.

PAY ATTENTION NOW... IMPORTANT STUFF COMING UP NEXT!!!
(Definitely exam material here!)

Things to know about Jim that are *different than Bob*:

1) Jim **HAS TO** know that you are listening to him (by doing what he says and NOT ignoring his messages) ***at least a couple of times a day,*** **EVERY SINGLE DAY OF YOUR LIFE!** (He's like totally insecure... ish – in a

control-freak kind of way). If you try to ignore him, he **WILL** keep messaging you over and over and over and over until you respond and if you still don't, he **WILL** call you up and talk to you or even yell at you and **WILL** eventually MAKE you to do what he wants you to do regardless of your objections. He doesn't use a cell phone like Bob; he uses a land-line[26]. This means that ***he can and he will keep going on and on for as long as it takes*** to make you do what wants you to do.

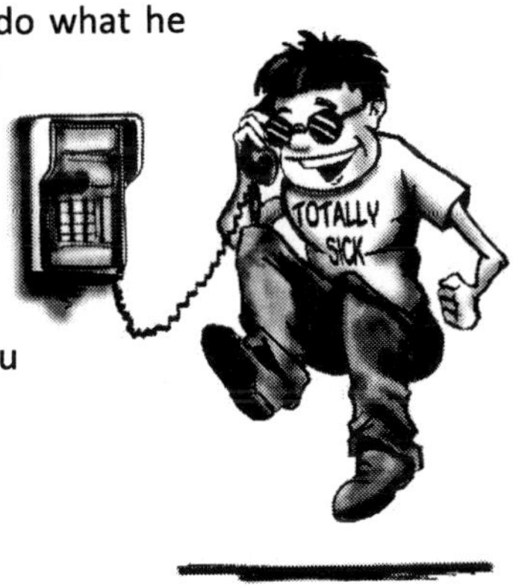

2) He's ***SHORT-SIGHTED*** when it comes to time and he ***can't really see stuff that's far away*** (in the future) unless it's **HUGE**.
3) He's ***SINGLE-MINDED*** which means that he is always very focussed on that thing that he wants you to go get... but what it also means is that he can ***ONLY FOCUS ON ONE THING AT A TIME***. In other words, he has to stop focussing on one thing if he starts focussing on something else.
4) He's not exactly lazy per se... but if he can, he will avoid having to work. He is always trying to come up with the easiest way to get the most Dopamine for your brain (the way that takes the least amount of effort for the biggest payoff).
5) He's stubborn and very strict about his job description which is ***making you Go Get Good Stuff***! This job description has 2 important implications:

[26] An old-fashioned kind of phone that plugs into the wall of your house and is attached by a cord... so it doesn't use batteries. *(Seriously!!!)* ... *(Ask your parents if you don't believe me!).*

i. **Everything on his *Good Stuff* list is considered to be equivalent ... interchangeable.**[27] This is why when you're having a great time at a concert/sport/activity, or you are playing a computer/video game you are hooked on, you don't feel hungry and 'forget' to eat. Because your brain is being flooded with Dopamine, it doesn't actively *want/crave* it since it is already getting it. Jim thinks you just ate because you did just get something on that list of *Good Stuff.* It's the same reason why smoking often makes people not feel hungry and also the reason why when they try to quit, they crave sweets and eat a lot more; Jim has to find replacement sources of Dopamine for the brain otherwise the craving is too intense to resist. The only differences between things on the list of *Good Stuff* is how much Dopamine it releases in your brain and how much effort will it take to get it.

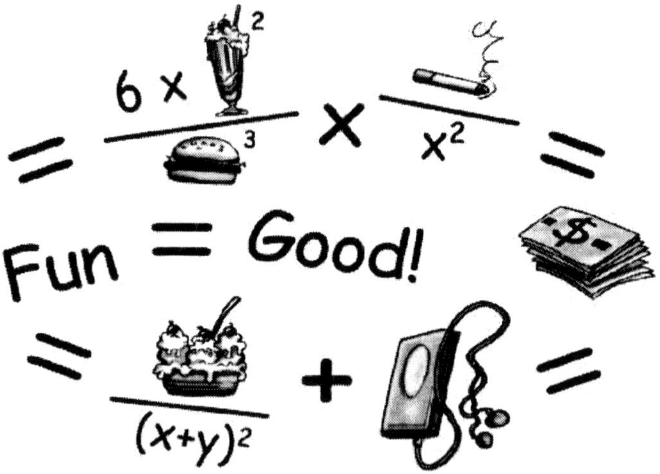

ii. Jim only cares about the *act of getting*, **NOT** the *state of having.* In other words, once he gets something, he quickly

[27] For the Math-brained people, another way of saying this is: food=smoking=music=video games=MSN=socializing=fun=sex=weed=chocolate=warm=**Dopamine**.

stops caring about it![28] ***He doesn't want (isn't activated/turned on by) what's already his! He only cares about (is activated/turned on by) what he's going to get next!*** For Jim, life really is... **all about the chase!!!**

6) He's very ***PERSISTENT AND DETERMINED***. At the end of the day, no matter what, one way or another, **Jim is always going to win and get his dopamine!** [29]

There is one last thing that you should know about Jim and Bob and it relates to what happens when both of them are messaging you, calling and talking to you and trying to get you to listen to them at the same time. If Bob and Jim are both suggesting that you do different things, you will generally try to make them both happy, if possible. If however, Bob is telling you to do one thing and Jim is telling you to do EXACTLY THE OPPOSITE, **Jim is going to win**. Jim knows that all he has to do is keep talking to you (keep you from being completely convinced by Bob) until Bob's cell phone dies, then he's got you all to himself (unless Bob is TONS LOUDER and more convincing and makes you act right away, before his battery dies).

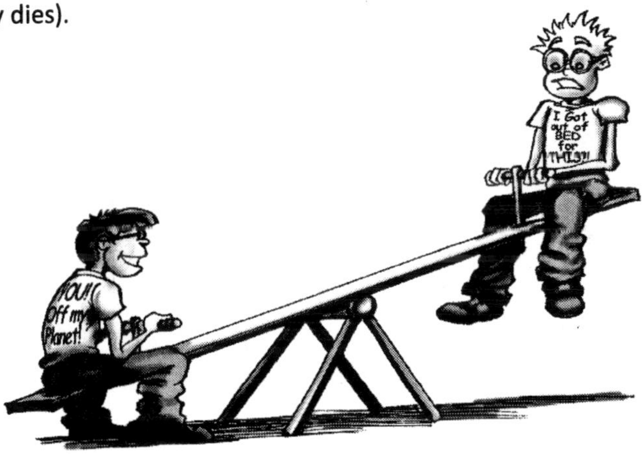

[28] This is the reason why your favourite things (songs, foods, people) eventually stop being your favourite things when you have it (listen to the song, eat the food, hang out with the person) constantly (i.e. it's basically 'yours').

[29] We have to eat or else we will die! And that's the most basic reason he exists – to make us eat.

Do you remember watching cartoons? Do you remember when one of the characters would be faced with a choice and suddenly, a little cartoon angel and a cartoon devil would pop out to sit on their shoulders and would take turns telling them what to do? The little angel would always be telling them to do the *right* thing – not break the rules, not steal the cookie, clean up the room, watch out for something. And do you remember what would happen when the little devil disagreed with the little angel? How they would solve that conflict? Remember??? The little devil would whip out his pitchfork and start beating the crap out of the little angel 😈.

That's kind of how 'Society' understands these two drives except that it's not quite right. You see, in the cartoons, the little angel was always telling them to do **good** things and the little devil was always telling them to do **bad** things. But in reality, the Harm-Avoidance Drive (little angel or Bob) and the Pleasure-Seeking Drive (little devil or Jim) are neither good nor bad... they just are. Either one can make you do *good* things **OR** *bad* things. To them, **the ends *ALWAYS* justify the means**. As far as they are both concerned, the only thing that's *'good'* is if they did their job (fulfilled their Prime Directive) and the only thing that's *'Bad'* is if they failed to do their job.

But the cartoons were right about one thing... at the end of the day, the little devil (Jim) always wins! 😈 😈 😈

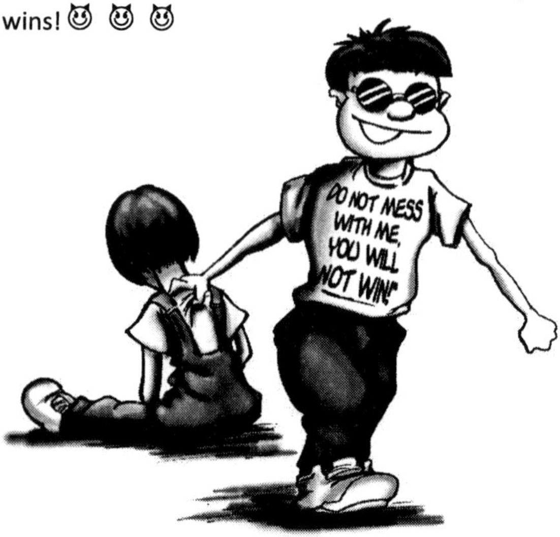

Chapter Somewhere Between Chapters 4 and 5

Interlude

insert cheesy elevator music here

Now that you know what these two drives do and how they work, you need to understand ***how*** they actually communicate with us. As you know, you don't really ***"hear"*** two distinct *voices* in your head; that's the analogy.

"  ?"

... Not again.... What? No! ...

Sometimes, once Logic and Reason develop, because we are aware of these instructions (thoughts) coming from somewhere and we know they are not from *'us'*, we conceptualize those two drives as being kind of like "*voices*" in our heads telling us to do things. Sometimes ***'WE'*** are even aware of the arguing back and forth that goes on between Jim, Bob and ***'US'***.

"  ?"

... No... Jim and Bob don't play Scrabble with you...

"  ?"

What do you mean they cheat???

"  !"

... OK....

"  !!!"

Well, that certainly explains a lot...

"  !?!"

I don't think that what you are hearing in your head is...

"  !!!!"

... OK, fine... that what you are hearing from the invisible baby stroller behind you... that's not Jim and Bob.

"  !?!"

... What?... Mathilda??? ... ...

"  !!!"

OOOOKAY then... SECURITY!!!!!

Back to the punch line. The way that these two parts of our brain communicate with us is through our ***THOUGHTS*** (this is how they message us – they make a thought pop into our heads [onto that screen in our brains]) and our ***FEELINGS*** (this is the point at which they have to call us on the phone to talk to us). When we ***feel*** something (any type of feeling at all), that '**feeling**' means that either Jim or Bob have got us on the phone and are talking to us. When these two parts of our brain '***talk***' to us, what our conscious brain '***hears***' is what humans refer to as the experience of having a ***feeling*** – we *feel like doing 'something'*. The *'something'* is what they are telling us to do while the ***feeling*** is equivalent to the sound of their voice through the phone and the *intensity of that feeling* is equivalent to how loud they get when they are talking to you.

Jim's voice is most often heard by your brain as *positive feelings* (**love**, lust, **happiness**, contentment, satisfaction, pride, **confidence**, excitement, etc.) though he does sometimes use a voice that you hear as negative feelings (**anger** [because you aren't getting something you want – which is about 95% of all anger in the world], irritation, envy, **jealousy**, etc.). Bob's voice is most often heard by our brain as *negative feelings* (**fear**, **guilt**, **shame**, feeling bothered, feeling unsettled, **nervousness**, **humiliation**, **worry/anxiety**, **jealousy**, anger [because you are being threatened and have to fight back to survive – which is about 5% of all anger in the world], etc.). Sometimes these emotions are appropriate, are based on reality and make sense (there really is a good reason you should feel angry/scared/guilty/worried) but equally, sometimes, they are completely inappropriate and make no sense at all (there really is nothing that actually happened, nothing that you actually did that should make you feel that way).

It is important to remember though that these two drives are there to make our lives easier – so that we don't have to *think* about every single thing that we do every day. Life would be too hard and too time consuming if we had to live that way. Because they DO make our lives easier and do most of the work for us, even after our Logic and Reason Center has developed, when Jim or Bob message us (i.e. put thoughts into our heads), we will usually just go right along with them and do what they suggest, rarely giving any *active, conscious* thought to, or analysis of what we are doing. Often, we will not even be fully aware of what it is that we did; we just run on automatic.[30]

If and when ***WE*** decide **not to** listen to them when they are just messaging us... and decide to do something else[31], even though it might not be that hard to do, it still takes an active effort to do it. It is a ***conscious choice*** that we have to make – to make our 'self' act differently. If, however, we stop 'thinking' about what we are doing (in other words, stop making a conscious choice) then we will quickly fall back into our old 'habits'[32]. But if we wait too long to try to make the decision to act differently... if they are already talking to us on the phone (i.e. when ***feelings*** come into the picture), then it will be much, **much** harder to '*think*' and to consciously override what those feelings are telling us to do. In other words, ***IF we*** *want to override Jim and/or Bob, it will always be easier to do it the minute we get the message (when the thought pops into our head). The longer we wait to go against them, the harder it will be*... eventually getting to the point where it will be impossible **not** to listen to them and obey.

30 This is basically what ***"bad habits"*** are.

31 in other words, make a choice **NOT** to run on automatic

32 patterns of behaviour

Chapter After the "Somewhere Between Chapters 4 and 5" Chapter

Growing Up – How Did "YOU" Get Here?

Monkey See, Monkey Do

Let's take a quick break and reminisce about the good old days... back when you were just a kid growing up... let's say from the day you were born until you were about 10 or 11ish. Do you remember those good old days well?

" ?"

What now... ... ...

" !"

No... you don't!!!

" !!!"

I don't care what you *think* you remember, I *know* you don't remember ***that***!!!

" !!!!!"

Oh Really? You think that ***that's*** why you're a good swimmer but are scared of small spaces???

" !"

No.... that ***wouldn't*** be the reason you have a fountain fetish....

" ?" " !!!" " !?!!?!"

OK... Other than Mr. Nutjob over there, how much of your childhood do you actually remember well? Of course, there are some things that you will remember. And the thing that all of those memories will have in common is that they will be about people or places or events which were very *emotionally intense*[33] for you as a child. But what about the *day-to-day* stuff that happened to you? How well do you remember that stuff?

---

[33] Which could be good emotions (i.e. proud, exciting, happy, etc.) or bad ones (i.e. terrified, angry, sad, embarrassed, etc.)

Kind of really hard to, isn't it? The reason that we don't remember much of our everyday life as kids is because the part of our brain that records that information is the Logic and Reason Center... and kids don't have it. Remember, it only starts to work properly around the time you start going through puberty.

The reason that I bring this up is because it's very important for you to recognize that when you were a kid (*and if you have any little annoying brothers and sisters at home, this applies to them too*), the only parts of your brain that controlled your behaviour were the two drives – Jim & Bob. All of your behaviour – everything that you did, at any given point in time, was done because of the balance of the relative volumes of these two drives.

How you behaved and what you did when you were a child, no matter what it was that you did, was simply ***because*** Bob and/or Jim told you to do it and you did it. And as I've just finished explaining in the previous chapters, **you had to listen to them and obey them**. Every action you took, everything you did was a direct result of what Bob and Jim had to say about what was going on in your world... about what you were experiencing in your life.

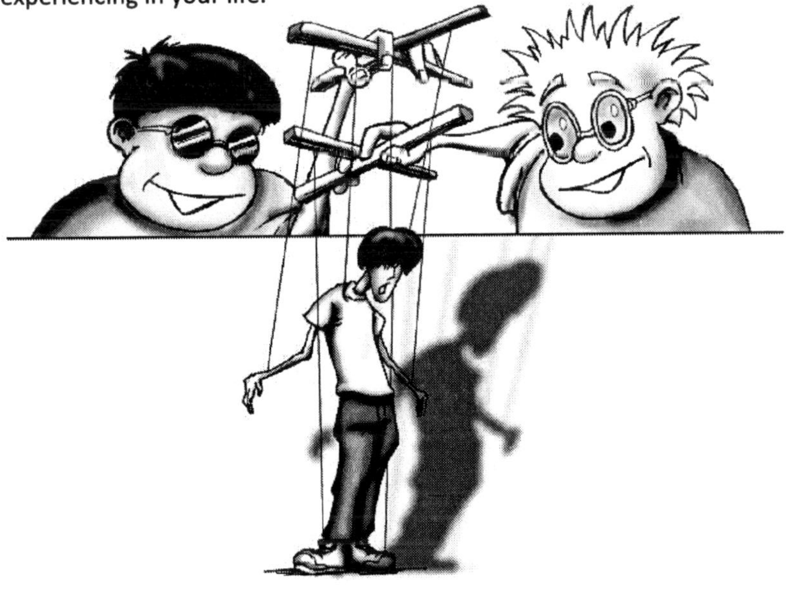

In other words, **YOU had no choice whatsoever.** ***YOU*** couldn't stop yourself from doing what they were telling your body to do because ***'YOU'...*** the part of the brain that is ***'YOU'*** (the Logic and Reason Center) didn't really exist yet... *the Logic and Reason Center wasn't online yet.*

Prior to the Logic and Reason Centre coming online, the kind of kid you were – whether that was a good kid, a bad kid, an angry kid or whatever – depended on only three things:

1) the characteristics of the physical body you were born into (i.e. Bob and Jim's work ethics),

2) Jim and Bob's lists of *Good Stuff* and *Bad Stuff* – in other words, what your personal experiences in life had taught you about what was good and what was bad and

3) what was going on around you at the time. And that's it. There was nothing else that mattered!

I'm going to discuss in a minute[34] in a little more detail what this means for you and why it matters in your life right now... because *knowing* this, *understanding* this and ***accepting*** this information is going to change your life!

Knowing is half the battle!

[34] *Or maybe longer... it depends on how fast you read!*

Chapter After the "Somewhere Between Chapters 4 and 5" Chapter – v. 1.2

Normal Childhood

How do our Brains Grow Up?

Monkey See, Monkey Do

The following applies to you... and everyone else too... assuming that you have a brain (*which obviously excludes THAT guy...*). When you were born, IF you had parents (or 'parent'-ish people) who took care of you (which basically means feeding you and keeping you warm), then by the time that you were about 18 months old, you had developed a ***hardwired bond*** or connection to those people. This *biological connection* that you developed doesn't depend on any shared genetics – it depends on who was there taking care of you and ensuring that you were fed, kept warm, kept safe and basically, kept alive for the first couple of years of your life. In other words, if you were adopted at or near birth, then this connection is to your adoptive parents, not your biological parents. If you were raised by your grandparents, then that connection will be to them.

"  ?"

... Yes...

"  ?"

Clearly if they were very intelligent monkeys, you would bond to them...

"  ?"

This explains a lot about you! **where the heck is security?????** For the sake of simplicity, I am going to refer to the people

"  !"

...yes, OK, or the highly intelligent monkeys... who cared for you in the first years of your life as 'parents'.

Once a child forms this bond to their parents, those parents will then be **very special** to that child. They will be seen as being the gods of that child's world. They will be the be-all and end-all. They will be seen by that child as perfect, infallible and all-powerful. As far as that child is concerned, there is nothing that they cannot do and nothing that they do not know.[35]

In children's eyes, parents are perfect, are never wrong and are completely trusted with anything and everything; literally even their lives.

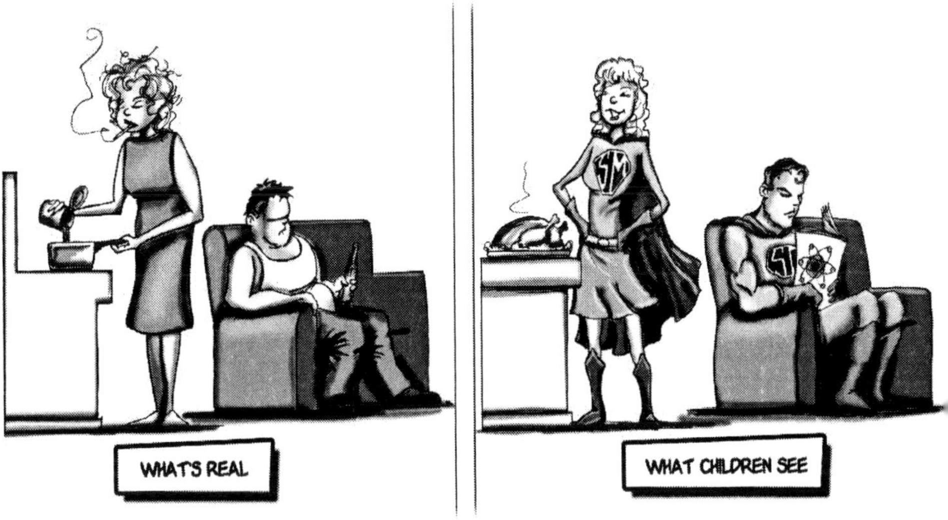

Part of the biological origins of this bond comes from the fact that Humans are a herding species.

WHAT THAT MEANS IS THAT BECAUSE WE'ZE ALL GOTS EARS... AND THAT MEANS THAT WE CAN HERD REAL GOOD EH!...

... 😳 😵 ...

Or maybe what it *really* means is that we are hard wired to collect in groups or clusters of individuals (like sheep, cows, deer, fish, ducks, dogs, horses and any other animal that seeks out others of its species to be near). Our parents are the first group or herd which we are exposed to and are therefore the first group into which we try to integrate[36] ourselves.

[35] Parents = 😇😇😇 = PERFECT

[36] join or become a member of

And as those of you who have memorized the Webster's Dictionary know, the definition of a herd is "a large assemblage of like things" or in plain English (applying it to people), "a bunch/group of people who are all alike/the same".

" !"

" !"

What do you mean you haven't memorized it? ... I thought everybody did that for fun on Friday nights... don't they?

NOPE... THAT'S JUST YOU BABY... ALL CURLED UP WITH A DICTIONARY WHILE I'M OUT PARTYING !!!

Oh Yeah?!? ... And if you're the other split of my personality, how exactly did you do that while my body was in bed wise guy???... DUH... ... ...

OH... IF ONLY YOU KNEW... ... ... DIDN'T YOU EVER WONDER WHY YOU NEVER WOKE UP IN THE SAME PLACE YOU THOUGHT YOU WENT TO SLEEP IN???

... but ... mom and dad said that I just used to sleep walk... a lot... every... week... end... ... ... w ... oh crackers[37]... just... just... go away!!! ... ...

As you know, the first step in joining or becoming a part of a group – any group – is to become like the other members of that group. We show that we belong to a 'group' by changing how we act, look, talk and think so that we are like them. And, believe it or not, this is exactly what we are hardwired to do at birth. First we identify the group and its leaders [our parents], and then we start mimicking them, copying them, and becoming like them. From the time we are born until around 10 or 11 (before our voices crack and our bodies start to bulge in weird places) we

[37] crap

automatically, without ever even thinking about it, walk like them, talk like them, dress like them, and act like them. Because we need to be completely accepted by them – at that age, our lives literally depend on it – we worship them, pretend to be them, and do everything in our power to try to grow up to be... **JUST LIKE THEM**.

And it doesn't stop with just walking and talking and dressing and acting like them; the most important thing that we end up doing just like them is ***thinking***. We mimic the way they ***think***; what they value and what they believe about the world. ***Before we hit puberty, we believe whatever it is that our parents believe***.

If our parents are Muslim and teach us about their beliefs, then we will believe Muslim beliefs. If our parents are Catholic, or Protestant, or Jehovah's Witnesses, we will believe whatever it is that they teach us about what Catholics or Protestants or Jehovah's Witnesses believe. If our parents are vegetarians or vegans or environmental activists or sexist or racist or white supremacists, we will be too. As children, we have no choice! We always grow up believing what our parents taught us about life and the world around us (remember... ... ... we trust them completely!!!). We will value what they value. We will believe what they believe. We will think what they think because, as children, we are incapable of 'thinking for ourselves'. We will see the world the same way that they see it – through their eyes. We are biologically designed to try to become small versions of them.

"!"

Yes, you are right! Sometimes, they don't *tell* us anything directly and sometimes, they even explicitly tell us *not* to be like them. But unfortunately, what they *tell* us really isn't that important. The most important way in which they teach us these things is by modelling them for us. We learn about life mostly by watching them. We mimic their behaviour long before we even become aware that there are reasons/meanings/beliefs behind what they do.[38]

What they do... how they act... their behaviours... ***these*** are the things that inform us of what they believe, much more powerfully than if they had simply *told* us what they believe. If our parents are clean freaks or Obsessive-Compulsive, if they have a temper, get angry a lot, scream or hit (us or others...), if they are passive and incapable, if they are scared or worried about germs or people or spiders or bugs and avoid them or hide or scream and freak out... we will grow up doing the same things and believing that these behaviours are OK (... and not just 'OK'... but something that ***we should be doing too***). We will believe that the way to solve conflict is to scream or hit, or that those fears are justified and those things are dangerous ...

BUT THEY ARE!!!

No one asked you... shut up! ... ... You!!! Yeah, you! ... ...

... ...

OK, you can continue now. He won't be giving you any more trouble!

... ...

Uhhhh... And who are you??? ...

You really don't want to ask that question... ... because If I told you the truth, then I would have to kill you... ... Just call me Mr. Pookie. ...

Ummmmm... this is getting a little bit weird... ... ... one sec... ... let me take my meds... ... ...

OK. ... That's better. (I hope) Now... ... where was I...???...

---

[38] For example, we copy them and learn to recite the Lord's Prayer long before we even know what a 'prayer' is or who 'the Lord' is.

Monkey See, Monkey Do

"!!!"

Nice try…

"!"

OK. Right!

As children, even with no understanding of what the behaviours mean, we will simply mimic their behaviours and make them a part of the behavioural patterns of our lives. And because they were the first things that we learned, ***those basic behavioural patterns will be the hardest of any to change or step away from***.

Of all the things that you learned about life and the world from your parents, the most important thing that you learned from them isn't any of the things that I just mentioned[39]. The **most important thing** you learned from your parents was about

TELEVISION… AND HOW TO USE THE REMOTE!

… No… It's You!

WHAT? WHO? HUH?

You!

WHAT ABOUT ME?

NO… not 'you'… … "You"!

WHAT THE… ARE YOU SMOKING THOSE WALKING CUCUMBERS AGAIN?

Oh for the love of… … You!!! … '***YOU***'!!!

YOU LOVE ME NOW??? ARE YOU GUYS SEEING THIS TOO? I THINK HE'S LOST IT COMPLETELY! TIME FOR ME TO TAKE OVER!!!

---

[39] It's not religion or politics or eating habits or how to treat others.

Not so fast there Mr. Black… did you forget about me?

WHO YOU? ME? NO… NO … MEDS KICKING IN NOW….

Thanks Mr. Pookie.

No prob.  …

… Ummm …  *… but if the meds finally kicked in… then why are YOU still here?*

Who?

You!…

You who?

… … …

… BRB…

We are experiencing technical difficulty – Please hold…

We are experiencing technical difficulty – Please hold…

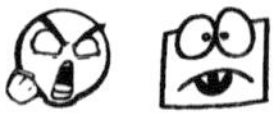

We are experiencing technical difficulty – Please hold…

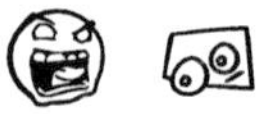

We are experiencing technical difficulty – Please hold…

Monkey See, Monkey Do

We are experiencing technical difficulty – Please hold...

We are experiencing technical difficulty – Please hold...

... ... 

We are no longer experiencing technical difficulty – You may now continue.

As I was saying, the **most important** thing that you learned from your parents has to do with ***"YOU"* ...** who ***"YOU"*** are. What you start out believing about yourself is what you saw mirrored in your parent's eyes. You believe that you are whatever your parents told *you* you were, and most of the information they give you and teach you about who you are is based on how they treated you (their behaviour and interactions with you as well as what they said directly to you).

A child whose parents are very permissive – in other words, they rarely correct them or say 'no' to them – grows up with a sense of entitlement, believing that everything they do is OK and above reproach. A child whose parents rarely set limits on them does not believe that they should have limits set on them by anyone (such as teachers or police or society). A child whose parents rarely complimented them grows up believing that they are not worthy of compliments. A child whose parents were very critical of them grows up believing that they are always wrong, that they can't do anything right, that no matter how hard they try, they will never be good enough.

Critical Parents

A 'critical' parent may not be what you think it is. Yes, obviously, if a parent calls their child an idiot or stupid or good-for-nothing, then they are being critical. If parents flat-out tell their child that he was a mistake, that their lives would have been better if she had never been born, that they can't wait for him to grow up and leave... so that they do not have to put up with her anymore, or if they flat out insult him, call her names, belittle him... then they are definitely being critical.

But what about if parents only notice or point out what's wrong with what a child has done? Or focus on the 10% missed rather than the 90% gotten right? Or spend their time with their kids correcting them and pointing out their mistakes, re-cleaning what their kids cleaned or redoing what their kids did? Well, yes, ***those*** parents are being critical too (and unfortunately, the reason *"why"* they did it, even if it was with good intentions, doesn't really matter that much).

If the majority of the interactions that a ***parent initiates***[40] ***with their children*** are negative – which basically means noticing what they're doing wrong, getting them in trouble, yelling at them, telling them what NOT to do or what to STOP doing – which would sound like an awful lot of:

- "Don't touch that!"
- "Stop picking your brother's nose! Pick your own!"
- "Leave the cat alone! Pets aren't chew-toys! "
- "Did you clean your room yet?"
- "Stop dragging your feet and **HURRY UP**! We've got to go!! The police are coming!!!"
- "Will you be quiet/stop yelling/making noise!"
- "Try not to be stupid/an idiot this time will you?"
- "How many times do I have to tell you ... the dishwasher is NOT A KITTY CAR WASH!!! The hair plugs up the drain!"
- "No, you can't bury him here!"

Or if parents simply don't interact much at all with their kids for whatever reason (workaholic, raised by a nanny, unable to because of their own physical/emotional limitations)... those parents are also being 'critical' parents.

---

[40] Doing something to get the child's attention focussed on them so that they can communicate with them.

Whether these parents know it or not, whether they mean to or not, their kids are going to grow up believing that they suck… that they screw up all the time… that they can never get it right… that they aren't and will never be *'good enough'*… that they are failures, bad kids, something to be fixed, something to be tolerated – all the while loving their parents to death and believing that their parents are the most awesome people in the world, trying to become just like them… and therefore feeling horribly guilty that their parents ended up with kids like them instead of the 'good' kids that their parents deserved.

Unfortunately, most of us (humans in the world) were raised with *'critical'* parents (to one degree or another[41]). And, unfortunately, we learn how to parent from our parents and our parents learned how to parent from their parents as well. Now, what this means is that your parents didn't know any other way to raise you! They simply raised/parented you in the same way that their parents raised/parented them. And, unfortunately, as every parent will tell you, kids don't come with an instruction manual[42].

Parents are only human and, despite what their kids think, they make mistakes… a lot of them. Unfortunately, kids don't have the ability to use logic and reason. As a child, you couldn't understand that your parents were only human, that they could make mistakes, that they might be wrong. You could not take into account the fact that they were stressed out or sick or tired or hung over or depressed or anxious or …

"  ?"

Yes, fine… or highly intelligent monkeys. The thought never crossed your mind that what your parents were telling you (either through their words or their actions) might not be what they really believed or might not be the really-for-real truth. You couldn't understand that some things might be

---

41 Obviously, some parents can be much, much more critical than others – which would mean that their kids would have much, much more of a problem.

42 *But I'm planning on changing that… it should be published soon - "The Kid's Instruction Manual - For Parents"*

their fault... that ***they*** made a mistake... that the ***reason they said or did what they did was because there was something wrong with them***. Your brain would not allow you to even consider that possibility. In kids' eyes, their parents are not mere mortals, prone to mistakes and lapses in judgement; they are like **Gods** – always right... perfect... able to do anything – leap tall buildings in a single bound, run faster than a speeding bullet, beat up *YOUR* dad!

Equally unfortunate is the fact that most parents never even think about this. Most parents don't realize how important they are to your world. They think that kids understand that they are tired or sick or cranky or might not really mean what they are saying. They make the mistake of thinking that kids think the same way that adults do; that kids know that people sometimes say things that they don't really mean when they are angry or drunk or stoned or sick or tired. They just don't get it – because no one has ever explained it to them.

Parents don't understand how a child could possibly worship them and love them so unconditionally... whether they ask for it or not, whether they like it or not, whether they deserve it or not, whether they are a good parent or a bad parent, even if they abuse you, hurt you, lie to you, ignore you completely or even walk out of your life for years. They don't understand that kids ***only*** understand emotions, not logic and reason. They don't know that you learn so much more from their emotional reactions and what they do than you do from what they say.

If only they knew what happened in your head when they got angry and screamed at you and told you that they were sick and tired of you or of looking at you or hearing you... that you were a rotten kid or a pain in their __ or a little __ ... or that they wished you would just go away or leave them alone or get out of their face or had never been born.[43] Things like that *cause* children to *feel bad.* And unfortunately, because of those events and hearing those things, their little Bobs often go and add something else to their database of *Bad Stuff* – **them**.

[43] *The things that some parents will say to their kids about them are some of the most disturbing things that I hear about in my practice.*

And unfortunately, ***these*** are the things that people will remember most from their childhood.

And then comes puberty... that magical time in life when your body starts to get weird on you, growing things that weren't there before like ...

"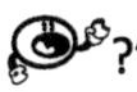?"

Yes!

"?"

That too!

"?"

Oh for crying out loud... are you for real???

"?"

... Oh... you are?

"?"

OMG... *OK... I really DID NOT need to see that...*

"?"

I'm sorry. I have no idea what it is. Go see a doctor or something!

"?"

I mean a surgeon - someone who can cut it off - not ME!

"?"

Yes; that's <u>DEFINITELY</u> not supposed to be there!

Monkey See, Monkey Do

So, yes, all of those things (*not that thing though... that's sick - and I don't mean the good kind of sick!*) grow and change but the **MOST** important part of your body that grows and develops is

"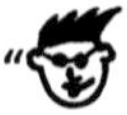!" ... ...

... *sigh*  ... ... well, guys might think so, but no, not that. ...

It's the ***NEW*** part of your brain[44] that can ***THINK***; the *Logic and Reason Center*... a.k.a. "Mini-U" (I'll introduce you to him in a second... or a week... depending on how fast you read). When it starts to grow, it changes your life forever and whether you like it or not, your world will never be the same again.

Now unfortunately, most adults in the world have no idea that this is happening – because they can't see your brain growing and changing. And because they don't know about it, they can't tell you about it – what to expect when it happens, why it is growing and changing, what to do with it, or how to use it. What adults **DO** tell you about are the external, physical changes that you go through (you know... "***THE***" talk that a lot of parents know they should have with their kids once they hit puberty...). And just in case your parents don't have that talk with you, society has decided that it is *so important* for you to know about what is going on with your body that they have put it in the school curriculum[45].

I'll tell ya, they (adult society) totally missed the boat on this one. Yes, they're right, it is important to know about the changes that happen in your body, but it is **WAY MORE IMPORTANT** for you to know about the changes that are happening in your brain!!! It's like getting a new car when you're 16 and in order to prepare you for the responsibility of owning and using your car for the rest of your life, your parents (or other adults at school) teach you how to put gas in the tank and how to turn the key to start it up. If they are real keeners, they might even teach you about how to change the oil, check the tire pressure and other maintenance things... but, they all

---

44 *the big brain, not the little brain guys...*

45 *Are they still using Bananas and cabbage leaves as the props?*

missed the boat because the problem is that *no one has bothered to teach you how to drive it!!!* ... let alone the *Rules of the Road*! So, I'm trying to fix that little oversight on their part right now! (Read on...)

That's why I'm writing this book for teenagers... I know that it doesn't take much to teach you how to drive at this stage in your life and I'm hoping that if enough people read this, then there will be a new generation of drivers out there that are good drivers [Generation 3 ... or 1 ... depending on how you look at it], confident in their ability to drive on this road we call life... and feeling comfortable behind the wheel of their car. I also believe that if enough people know the Rules of the Road (3 simple rules about life that you need to know[46]), then there will be fewer accidents, less tragedy, fewer struggles and break downs - less work for the EMS crews [that would be people like me who try to fix people up when they crash in life].

(What can we say... He's lazy and would rather not have to work for a living! 😆)

[46] *See Chapter 140 km/h (after Chapter 11)*

Chapter 5

Introducing... Mini-U!!!

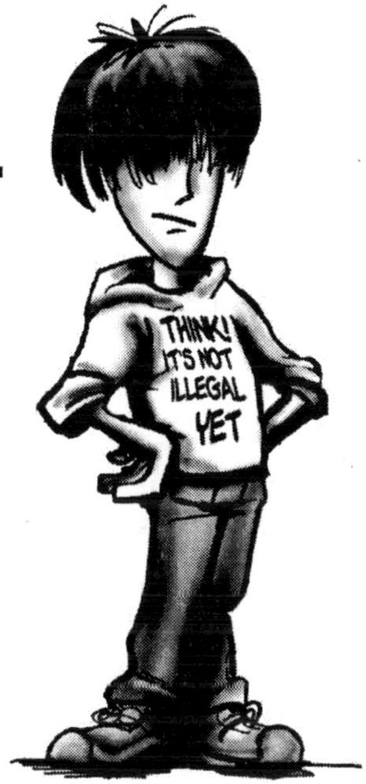

a.k.a.

The Logic and Reason Center

I Think I Can Think, Can You?

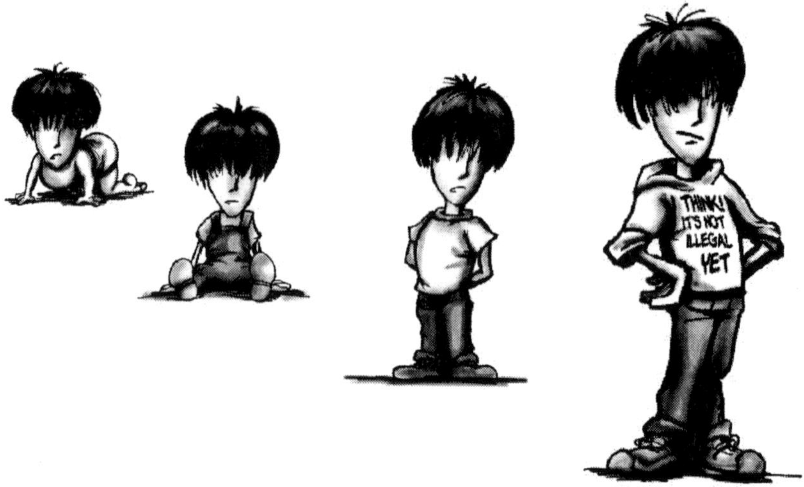

Now for the important stuff. The next part of the brain that I am going to talk about is the *'Logic and Reason Center'* or, as I like to call it, *"Mini-U"*. **It** is **THE MOST IMPORTANT part of the brain.** **It** is the ***'smart'*** part of the brain. Oh yeah... and it's also the part of our brain that holds *'us'*... the concept of "***Us***"... the thing that makes us who 'we' are – uniquely different from everyone else out there in the world. **It** is the part of our brain that makes up ***our*** thoughts, ***our*** ideas, and ***our*** values. **It**, more than anything else in our brains, bodies or lives, is what determines what ***our*** *'human experience'* is going to be like. **It** is what makes us *individuals*. **It** is *'who we are'* – which is why I call it "Mini-U".

For the purposes of the analogy I have been using, think of this third part of your brain as being a little mini version of **you** (... *can you guess how I came up with the name "Mini-U"?* ☺). Mini-U has a voice and volume of his own and, together with Jim and Bob, makes up the three 'voices' or behaviour-controllers in our heads.

Unlike the two drives, Jim and Bob, the Logic and Reason Center – Mini-U – is well known. Every normal adult and every normal teenager knows about this part of the brain. They are very familiar with it (*though they might not use it that much*) and talk about it and discuss it quite regularly in their everyday lives. I'm ***sure*** you've heard people talking about it and have even talked about it yourself (though you might have used different terms). What everyone else calls this part of the brain is '***common sense***'. This is part of our brain that '***thinks***' – that *understands what is real and what is not real*. **It** is the part of the brain that recognizes the importance of your toenails in decision making and is the reason why cows orange us people with brown hair shouldn't part their cars to the up.

It is the part of our brain that *analyzes and understands the world we live in*. **It** is the part of your brain that just finished saying "Huh? What?" when you read the last sentence of the previous paragraph (*and maybe even made you re-read it to be sure that you read it right*). *It is the part of our brain that decides if something **'MAKES SENSE'**!* It is intricately involved in the human experiences of 'understanding' something, 'thinking about' something, 'deducing'[47] something, and 'being confused' about something.

So then, how does Mini-U work? What does Mini-U **do**? Essentially, Mini-U is the problem-solver in our brain. He uses information to solve problems – to find fact-based solutions to the problems and obstacles that we encounter in our every-day life. Mini-U is what gives us the ability to go beyond our Drives' programming, to adapt to new situations, to learn new information and use this information to apply Logic and Reason and *think* about what makes sense to do in any given situation (based on what we know to be true). This then allows us to act in a way that makes sense so that we can achieve our objectives.

The way that Mini-U works is similar in some ways to the way Jim & Bob work. Mini-U starts out by acquiring information – learning '*about*' or learning '*what*'[48], or learning why – and entering it into his list of '*Stuff I Need to Know*'. In other words, Mini-U first collects information, evidence, proof, 'knowledge' or facts then takes all of this information and puts it into a big, cross-referenced database (database = big encyclopaedia in head). In order to create this database, Mini-U analyzes our environment (making note of all of our sensory data – everything that we see, smell, hear, taste and feel), and then takes that information and copies it into **his**

[47] This is what Sherlock Holmes did.

[48] Learning '*how to*' is not nearly as important to Mini-U.

database. He tries to write as much stuff as he can into his database in order to be able to do better at his job.

The more stuff he learns, the more he knows and therefore the better he can be at his job. He doesn't care about whether information is good or bad or neutral or anything; he'll put anything in it and tries to put as much stuff as he can in there. His database is a constantly growing collection of '**facts**'. What Mini-U considers a "**fact**" is anything that we actually saw/heard/experienced ourselves or something that we were told about by someone that we trust (*if Mini-U believes that what they are saying is true and factual, he will write that information into the database almost as if we had experienced it ourselves*) ... **unless** we have experienced something that contradicts it. (*Did I mention yet that 'personal experience' is the most powerful way to add stuff to any of the three databases?*)

The cool thing about Mini-U is that, while Jim and Bob are stuck using little pictures of things pasted onto a long piece of paper for their databases, he gets a super-deca-octo-quadratic-double cored super-computer to use for his database. Once there's enough information in that database, he comes online and starts learning how to use his awesome database. His job then becomes the ongoing collection of information to continue to build that database and also the comparison of all incoming information with what's already in that database.

This process...

– Comparing new information with what we already know from what we were taught and what we have experienced –

is what it means to try to "*Make Sense*" of something.

Now, if you were awake and paying attention back around chapter 2, you might remember me saying that this part of the brain is not present in children. The basic hardware for it is there, but it doesn't start working the way it's supposed to until you hit puberty, which is when it *starts* to mature. In a lot of ways, it's like the body's sex organs – they are there in kids **but** they don't work the way they are supposed to until puberty when they start to change from their 'immature' states to their mature, functional states. When I say that kids can't '*think*', it's like saying that kids can't make babies – yes, they have the parts that will eventually be able to do that, but no, they don't work yet. When we are kids, all that Mini-U can really do is collect that information. He doesn't know what to do with it yet. He can't really analyze it, compare it or understand it... but he can put it in there, so that's what he does.

Mini-U starts to mature (learn how to use the information rather than just collect it) around the time we hit puberty and he continues to develop and grow in strength and ability (i.e. how finely he can dissect down information to its component parts, how quickly he can analyze and compare incoming information and how thorough[49] a comparison he makes) during our teen and young-adult years. How well Mini-U does at collecting and analyzing information is essentially what we refer to as 'intelligence'.

Mini-U knows that you can't build a house if he doesn't know what a house is made of and you can't cook food if he doesn't know what **heat** is or how to use it. So, in order to help prepare us for being an adult, Mini-U starts building and organizing our database for us to use around the same time as we start building our new adult bodies. The reason that this part of our brain develops and matures at the same time as our bodies do – when transitioning from child to adult – is that it is critically important to use it properly as an adult. It benefits us and makes it much more likely that we will survive 'life'.

You see, as an adult, we *have to be able to think*, problem-solve, and then *adapt* our behaviour based on what's in our immediate environment. In

[49] How carefully he compares it to what's already in there and how many things he compares it to.

other words, as adults, **we need to be able to act in ways that make sense!!! Even if it means going against what our Drives are telling us to do.** This ability to override our drives to any extent is what sets us apart from the rest of the animals in our world.

If you understand everything I've explained about the Logic and Reason Center so far, then it should be obvious that ***IT IS THE PART OF OUR BRAIN THAT IS SUPPOSED TO BE IN CONTROL OF OUR BEHAVIOUR!!!***

Once we grow up, we all *expect* that everyone else is using this part of their brain to control their own behaviour. ***We expect other people to act in a way that makes sense.*** We know that *our world makes sense* and, therefore, in order to be part of our society, our behaviour is supposed to make sense too – in other words, be consistent with reality. Our survival and the survival of our species depend a great deal on our ability to do this. Consider the language that we use if this isn't what's happening; terms like 'nonsense'[50], 'irrational'[51], 'unreasonable'[52], 'senseless'[53] are not flattering. In fact, to refer to someone using those terms would be very insulting.

When someone acts in a way that makes no sense at all, it bothers us. For example, say that one day, your best friend showed up at your house wearing a tutu over top of a clear garbage bag, holding a toilet plunger in one hand and clutching a potato to his ear, did not recognize you but pushed past you and knelt down in front of your pet Chihuahua and called it by your name and started talking to it as though the dog was you, telling him to run and hide in the basement because Emperor Zorgon's invasion of earth is going to happen in 3 hours. Then he rambles on explaining to your Chihuahua that he knows this for a fact because he happened to overhear the invasion plans coming out of the alien communication device that they had cleverly disguised as a potato... and he seriously believed this...

---

[50] a.k.a rubbish, garbage, drivel, gobbledygook

[51] a.k.a illogical, foolish, ridiculous, absurd, silly

[52] a.k.a unfair, unwarranted, uncalled for, perverse

[53] a.k.a stupid, foolish, unwise, idiotic, ridiculous

We call that kind of behaviour "**crazy**". And as you know, *'crazy'* people are generally not allowed to roam around and mingle with the rest of us – it makes us 'normal' people (*and I use that term very, very loosely considering some of the people here...*) very, very, **very** uncomfortable.

"  ?"

No, I'm not referring to myself!!! ....

Any social or cultural group has, as a basic premise, the idea that any clearly abnormal behaviour (behaviour not based on very basic logic and reason[54]), is a sign of something being very wrong with that person. In our modern culture, we see it as evidence of a *'mental illness'* but in other times, and in other cultures, it's been seen as evidence of other things – like possession by evil spirits, being mind controlled by alien celery stalks, mental deficiency punishable by death, being cursed by the gods – all of which are not considered 'good', but rather, something people should avoid.

When Mini-U comes online and matures, he has one critical, fundamental, unwritten rule he uses when analyzing information. We all know it and fundamentally understand it, and for the most part accept it and apply it all the time. That rule is: **"IF IT DOESN'T MAKE SENSE, THEN IT'S NOT REAL!"** Remember, when you were a kid, you did not have Logic and Reason as a functional process in your brain. Your world did not need to make sense, and could be magical and full of fantasies that you believed were real. The development of Logic and Reason is why, even if no one ever said a thing about it, by the time kids become teenagers, (assuming they have a normal brain) they *know* the truth about Santa... and the Easter Bunny ... and the Tooth Fairy... and start to wonder about their parents.

Before the development of Logic and Reason, there is no awareness of the rule that things need to make sense in order to be real or true. In fact, before Mini-U comes along, kids have no concept of what it means to *'make sense'*. Oh sure, they can nod their heads and agree with their

---

[54] Mind you, historically, this criteria was ignored – thus many scientists and 'thinkers' were put to death because they tried to convince people to think more.

parents when they are asked if something makes sense or not but if you ask them what it means to 'make sense', they have no idea. Because 'making sense' means being analyzed by the Logic and Reason processing center and having Mini-U decide that it is consistent with all of the other information in the database – therefore, giving that piece of information his 'OK' as being logical and reasonable.

Mini-U's job takes a lot of energy. It's hard work. While Jim and Bob get to take a snapshot picture of stuff and paste the pictures into their databases, Mini-U has to enter it all in, while at the same time, organizing it as he goes and comparing it to everything else that's already been accepted as 'true'. Unfortunately, for any information to be useful to Mini-U, it *has to be* organized and cross-referenced and checked for accuracy/validity (like a quality-control person checking stuff that comes off the assembly line). Think about it... even if you could have all the information about everything in the world written down somewhere, it would still be useless unless you knew how to find specific information you want, when you needed it. It's like the Internet – just about everything you would ever want to know on a subject is there... somewhere. Now, if you know how to find what you are looking for quickly and easily, then it's a **useful** source of information; otherwise, it's just a jumbled, useless mess.[55]

Because Mini-U's job is demanding (when he is putting information into the database AND when he is searching through and retrieving information from the database) sometimes he misses stuff or decides to ignore stuff. Sometimes, he only jots it down in point-form without really doing his job of checking for accuracy and cross-referencing it properly (i.e. understanding it), especially when there is a lot of information coming at him at the same time[56] or when he is already busily working to find and retrieve information to give to you.[57] So, given that Mini-U is the part of

---

[55] *I mean seriously... how useful is it to know that you 'know' something (a word, a name, a phone number, etc.) if you can't 'think of it' when you need it?*

[56] Mini-U: **"Whoa... slow down, I can't *understand* what goes where, when, why and with whom when I'm being bombarded by information from everywhere all at once!"**

[57] Mini-U : **"sorry, can't enter data right now... I'm busy looking something up for you!"**

the brain that is most responsible for storing, accessing and retrieving information – our 'knowledge' about the world – can you figure out what happens to a lot of information when Mini-U isn't 'online' yet?

"  ?"

What????? NO! Why on earth would your head implode???

"  !"

*... *sigh**  *Please... please.... Just think about it for a second... Do you see kids walking around with their heads imploding??? Remember what I said just a couple of minutes ago about Mini-U and Kids?*

"  ..."

No, huh.... hmmmm... Well, that explains a lot.

" 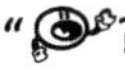 ?"

'That' is the fact that you don't remember me saying that... You see, 'memory' is information that was: a) encoded by Mini-U and b) retrieved by Mini-U.

"  ?"

Exactly! That's exactly why you can't really remember your every-day, normal childhood experiences very well (except for those experiences that were very positively or negatively emotional that are in Jim and Bob's databases). But once you hit grade 7 or 8, you start being able to remember all sorts of useless stuff about what happened to you – everyday boring stuff.

Now, what about the situation where Mini-U is online but isn't the one in control and is being actively excluded because Jim or Bob is in the driver's seat and screaming,[58] and Mini-U is completely drowned out? Same thing! It's hard to remember exactly what you said or did during those times when Jim and/or Bob are screaming at you (you are enraged or distraught or terrified or otherwise overwhelmed by your emotions). It's also just as hard to think and pull information out of storage too

"?"

Yes, that's exactly why sometimes, when you've been in a situation like that, "it's all just a blur..."

Keep in mind that while Mini-U is analyzing the world, he is also analyzing our own behaviour... and identifying when what *we* are doing makes no sense at all. Our awareness of this part of our brain is often like a real voice – not just like the analogy of the Drives but a much more distinct and recognisable one... it's ***'Us'***, talking to our 'self', commenting to our 'self', questioning our 'self', often even criticizing our 'self' (our actions and behaviours) because we *know* that we shouldn't be doing those things. Sometimes, we even tell ourselves or others that we don't '*want*' to do them... ***because*** we *know* better or because it makes no sense to do them or because of whatever...

Unfortunately, when we are growing up, we have to trust our '*feelings*' to guide us through life, because we have no choice. We don't have anything else to rely on. What this means is, when it comes to the battle for control of our behaviour, because Mini-U didn't join the game until much later, he starts out at a disadvantage (in terms of volume/strength) compared to Jim and Bob. But luckily, he does get progressively louder as he matures and grows and, most importantly, the more he plays the game and competes with Jim and Bob in order to control our 'self'.

There is, however, a big problem with Mini-U's maturing process – *people don't know about it*. People don't actively recognize that this is happening. Unfortunately, people have never been told and weren't taught that there

[58] i.e. when you are in an intense emotional state.

is another player entering the game and that they are supposed to put as much energy and effort as they can into helping him develop, so that he can become as strong as he is supposed to be[59].

As a result of that ignorance... and also because the Drives have been there since Day One and people recognize them and know them well... and also because they can be really loud (their maximum volume is 10/10)... and also because people had nothing else to rely on for those 'internal orders' when they were growing up... and also because people are often told to... for all of these and other reasons, people (adults and teenagers) continue to trust their two Drives to direct their lives.

Have you ever heard someone say "Trust your feelings!"... ??? I hope not... even though you probably have... because that's the STUPIDEST thing I have ever heard!!!

"  ?"

... ...  ... ...  ... ...  ... ... *ok... I take it back... THAT is the stupidest thing I have ever heard...*

I hope that it's obvious by now that ***the idea that you should 'trust your feelings' is absolutely absurd!!!*** Why on earth would you trust something that often makes no sense at all and that cannot think or understand what's real? Sure, sometimes Jim and Bob might be right... but they might also be **wrong!!!** Mini-U, on the other hand, ***SHOULD*** be trusted and we ***SHOULD*** listen to what he's telling us to do; **especially if it is contradicting what our 'feelings' are telling us to do!!!**

When people are in an emotional state (angry, scared, anxious, sad, in love), then you know for a fact that they are not *'thinking'* clearly. And yes... this includes you too. When Jim and Bob are yelling at you, Mini-U has a very hard time getting a word in edgewise since he isn't anywhere near loud enough to be heard over them yet! Is a Daddy Long-legs really-for-real dangerous? ... Will a garter snake really-for-real kill us? Does it

59 loud enough to be able to override anything that Jim and/or Bob are saying to do when what they are saying makes no sense at all

really-for-real make sense to smoke? Are they really-for-real going to change for us just because we love them? Is he really-for-real not going to cheat on you again when he already has several times in the past? Can she really-for-real be trusted not to lie to you again? (*The really-for-real answer to all of those is "No!"...*). You cannot and should not trust your feelings!

DON'T TRUST YOUR FEELINGS...

TRUST YOUR THINKING!!!

It does not follow that, just because you feel a certain way, there MUST be something real giving rise to those feelings. This is simply not true. People often *feel* scared even though there is nothing to be afraid of; *feel* left out though they are clearly included; *feel* offended though there was no offensive comment made; *feel* like they can trust someone though there is no evidence that they should (and in fact, often a lot of evidence that says that they shouldn't); *feel* justified in their actions though there is nothing that would really justify what they are doing.

FEELINGS ARE NOT RELIABLE!!!

While they *might be right* (giving you instructions on how to act based on a real situation that *should* elicit such feelings/actions – i.e. feeling scared and wanting to run away from a bear in the woods or feeling angry because someone stole your wallet) they also *might be wrong* (giving you instructions on how to act based on an imagined/misperceived situation that *shouldn't* elicit such feelings/actions – i.e. feeling scared and wanting to run away from a Daddy Long-legs or feeling angry because someone driving in front of you is actually driving the speed limit).

And yet, people can't stop themselves from acting "crazy"... behaving in a way that makes no sense at all; jumping and screaming when they see a spider or a snake, continuing to smoke, staying in bad relationships, etc. For about 95% of adults (average, normal, functional adults), their Logic and Reason Center has maxed out at a volume level of about 5.84592 – able to override/ignore some of the stupid things that Jim and Bob tell them to do – but not all the time. Think of just about everyone you know; do some of them smoke? Do some of them do things that make no sense? Do they **only** do things that make sense? Do some of them get mad and lash out irrationally? Do some of them get stupid when they "fall in love"? Of the people you know, do any of them not fit into any of the above categories? Unfortunately, the vast majority of the world is stuck using only about 2.584592 parts of their brain[60] to control their lives.

The thing is... it doesn't have to be that way. If people had been taught when they were teenagers or young adults what was going on in their heads and were taught how to train their Logic and Reason Center (Mini-U) to help it develop and mature, then he could have gotten louder, louder even than Jim and Bob with a volume of 11 or 12, able to override and be louder than them no matter how loud they were screaming. They could have been people with *'will power'* – able to make themselves do what they know they should do, all the time – a generation of **3**s... or **1**s... depending on how you look at it. But once they are past their twenties, it's too late for them. Their brain is finished growing. It ***can't*** reshape itself and grow any more. Our brains stop growing up shortly after our bodies stop growing up. From roughly 25 years old on, as far as the shape and general size of our brain is concerned, it's pretty much all downhill from there.

---

[60] **1** (Harm Avoidance Drive) + **1** (Pleasure Seeking Drive) + **0.584592** (Logic and Reason Center) = **2.584592**

So then, how can ***you*** make Mini-U stronger? Louder? You need to ***use him to THINK about what makes sense to do as much as you can and as often as possible*** and then ***use him to try to OVERRIDE the instructions from Jim and Bob when what they are telling you to do makes no sense.*** *Focus on what you are doing and change that behaviour!* Force yourself to change it! Force yourself to do what makes sense. It's harder than you think! But it is this action (***"TRYING to override Jim and Bob to make yourself do…"***) that builds him up and makes him stronger and louder over time.

Just so you know what to expect though… *you will fail*! Time and time again, if you try to stop yourself from doing something or try to make yourself do something, *you will fail*. But the act of *'trying'* will, little by little, each time you try, make Mini-U will a little bit stronger, a little bit louder. And if you continue to do this every day, more and more, many times a day, you will start to win more often.

You have to keep in mind that building up Mini-U isn't something that will happen quickly – it will take about 18 months to 2 years of regularly working on this, working him out hard… trying to override/change what you are *doing*, in order to get Mini-U to a volume of more than 10. *There are no shortcuts when it comes to reshaping the hardwiring in your brain so don't expect that you can do it faster because you can't.* And don't get discouraged if a year from now, even after working on this every day, you are still losing to Jim and Bob a lot of the time; that's what's going to happen. There is no way around it. It's like anything else you try to learn in life – how to play the piano, the guitar, baseball, soccer, chess, dancing, etc. – it takes time (because your brain can only remodel itself at a certain rate) and practice and effort (you need to constantly tell your brain how you want it remodelled) in order to teach your brain how to do it well and become really good at it.

But if you do decide to do it... and join ***Generation 3... or 1... depending on how you look at it...*** you will be happy! Your life will be satisfying. *You*'ll be in control of *your* life and make it whatever *you* want it to be.[61]

Having a loud/powerful Mini-U is the single most important thing that protects you from having emotional problems in your life. It is the single biggest variable in being able to be "happy". Mini-U can tell you how to avoid all of those mistakes in life that everyone else has to suffer through. He can help you avoid the drama! He brings with him the ability to think and figure out how to succeed and win this game we call 'life'. If you don't believe me, try it! You'll see!

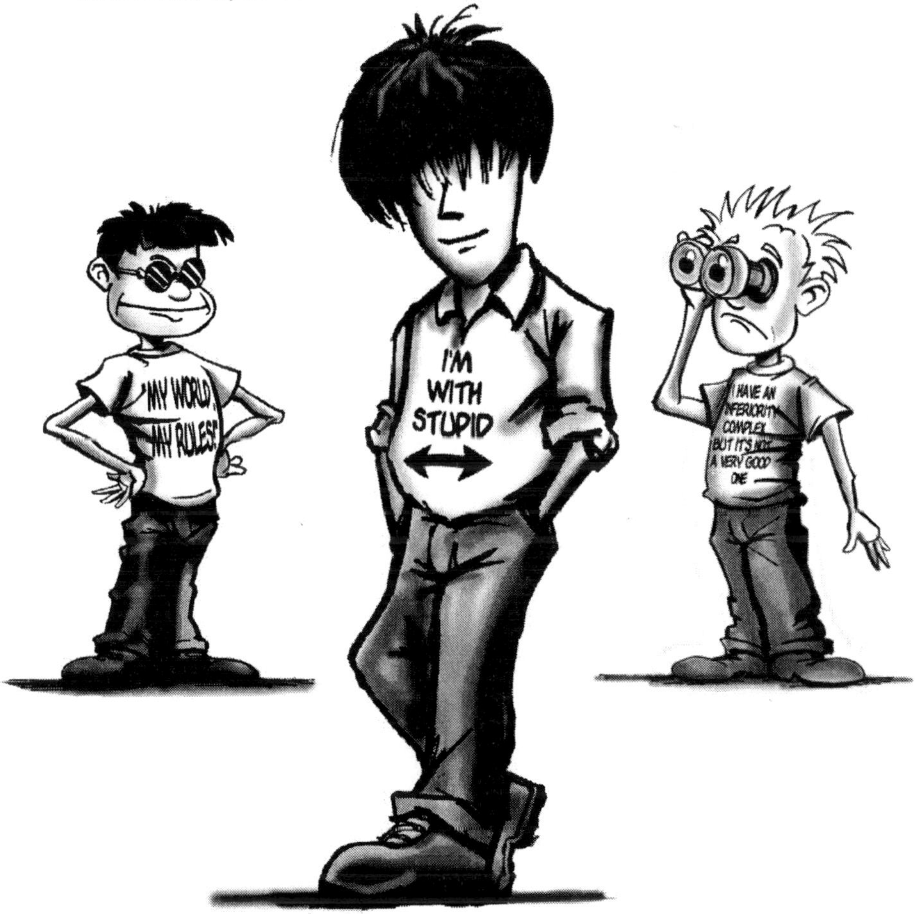

[61] ... *and I'll even send you a free T-shirt! It doesn't get much better than that!*

Chapter 5.1

One More Analogy

WARNING

This chapter is not for everyone!

Only read this chapter if you want to know more about how they all work ***AND*** *you understand a lot about computers & programming.*

Otherwise, you should just skip this part since it will probably just confuse you

<u>*Power Suits Are Fun!*</u>

I'm going to re-explain what I just did in the last 3 chapters using a different analogy – one more suited to the math-brained people – to help clarify the interplay between these 3 parts of our brains. Imagine, if you will, that our bodies are simply a great big complicated machine that is designed to be able to do just about anything – if it has the right program (software) and the right parts (hardware) installed. Think of it as being like a robotic powered cyborg suit made of skin, muscle and bones (instead of being made of just metal) with a super-computer integrated into it in order to run it – *like a fleshy version of the armoured suit worn by Iron-Person-who-isn't-a-woMan - freaking lawyers...*).[62]

When these suits are first built and come off the assembly line, in order to be able to work and do the most basic things (like stay turned on, walk, fly or shoot laser beams from its hands), it needs to have two hardwired, resident (always on) programs built into its Central Processing Unit (CPU).[63] These 2 programs are the "Power Management Program" (a.k.a. Jim) and the "Self-Preservation Program" (a.k.a. Bob).

The most important of these two programs is the **Power Management Program** [PMP] because it *<u>is dedicated to powering the suit</u>*; making sure there is always enough electricity in the suit's batteries for it to run. Because these suits are designed to be left **ON** all the time, part of the PMP's job is to constantly monitor the suit's power levels through the suit's *Internal Systems Monitors* (ISM) and also to constantly monitor the environment for usable power sources so that it can recharge its batteries when needed. In order to be able to do its job, the PMP is connected to two of the suit's primary functional systems[64]. It has a hard-wired data access connection to the *'Data Input Processing Unit'* [DIPU] and a hard-wired override built into the suit's *'Central Control Panel'* [CCP].

---

[62] *If you are confused as to what I'm talking about, there are several Hollywood movies that have examples of these kinds of "human suits": one of the aliens in "Men in Black" (1997), Dave in "Meet Dave" (2008), Iron Man in "Iron Man" (2008), everyone's surrogate in "Surrogates"(2009), Avatars in "Avatar" (2010).*

[63] This is the computer that controls the suit.

[64] hardware+software subunits – like a video card or a modem in a computer + the software to run it.

The Data Input Processing Unit [DIPU] is the part of the suit's computer that records and analyzes all of the information from the different input devices that are built into the suit (i.e. the audio data from the microphones located in its ears, the graphic data from the cameras built into its eye sockets, the data from the touch-pad sensors located on its cyborg skin, the temperature sensors, the built-in radar, the GPS navigation system, etc.).

The Central Control Panel [CCP] is the part of the suit's computer that controls every aspect of everything that the suit does at an incredibly detailed, micro-ordered level and is responsible for the execution of all commands. The way that the CCP works, in order to make it easy to control the suit[65] is the following: the CCP receives commands from the Power Management Program, the Self-Preservation Program and the user (a.k.a. Mini-U) and then interprets/breaks down those general commands into their component steps in order to execute the original command. For example, if the user or the Self-Preservation Program give the command "run", the CCP will take that command and translate/interpret it (break it down) to its component steps (which would include things like: flex left thigh at hip joint while also flexing left leg at left knee joint then shift balance of the suit's weight forward while extending at left knee joint and flexing at right ankle and extending rapidly at right knee joint and right hip joint and... you get the picture[66]) and then makes the suit do all of that stuff in a coordinated way. In other words, it makes the suit 'run'. Or another way to put it is that when the CCP is told ***WHAT*** to do, it then figures out ***HOW*** to do it and then makes it happen.[67]

The Power Management Program needs to have continuous access to all the data from the DIPU so that it can identify all possible sources of electricity in its immediate surroundings. It also needs to have a hard-wired override built into the CCP so that it can give the command to "seek and acquire electrical energy from... ..." whenever it needs to in order to recharge the suit's batteries.

---

[65] make it user-friendly

[66] I'll bet that you never realized just how complicated it is to do such simple things like walk, run, talk, sit down, stand up, throw a ball, catch a ball, etc...

[67] *hmmm... I probably should have just started with that explanation..*

Power Suits Are Fun!

Now, because this suit is so powerful and has so many functions, it's an energy hog and has a short battery life[68]. And, because its batteries are made of the latest Lithium-ion polymer and built right into the suit, the Power Management Program is programmed to never let the battery run out because, if it does run out completely, the suit will become non-functional… permanently. As a result of the suit's complete dependence on electrical power for functionality, the PMP has been given optional precedence over any and all other programs, functions or commands. In other words, it has the ability to override and highjack any of the functions of the suit in order to get recharged because, without any electricity in the batteries, the suit is going to shut down and be useless.

This ability to override and highjack the suit's functions is both *absolute* (it can highjack and override **anything**) and *progressive* (it will only highjack what it needs to get the job done – in other words, it is ***not*** all-or-none). The progression of the Power Management Program's degree of precedence is dependent on the current *Energy-Need Value* (ENV). The ENV is a numerical representation of the ***need/importance*** of electricity to the suit and is determined by the Power Management Program through a series of complex ***IF-THEN*** analyses of all the current data relating to power consumption, management and acquisition.

The equation used to determine the ENV is fairly consistent over periods of time but it will vary considerably over the life of the suit and will also vary between different suit models. Some of the more important factors that are analyzed when determining the suit's current ENV include (but are not limited to):

- The current level of electrical charge still left in the battery *****
- The battery's historical (last 2 weeks only) average charge level on which the unit was functioning (i.e. is the battery usually kept at 50% capacity, 75% capacity, 125% capacity… etc.) ****
- Recent energy expenditures ***

[68] how long it will be able to continue to run without recharging

- Predicted upcoming energy expenditures ***
- Currently identified sources of electricity in the immediate vicinity (along with the predicted amount of energy it should provide as well as the predicted energy expenditure that should be required to get it) ***
- The overall, historical, level of availability of electricity in its environment **
- And many other modifying variables that vary in importance. (from * to *****)

Of all the factors involved in the determination of the ENV, the current level of charge is the most critical and has the largest effect on the ENV. For example, if the historical average charge was 'high' (i.e. the suit was plugged in 20 hours a day), battery levels never dropped below 75%, sources of electricity were easy to find and the suit overall energy expenditures was low, etc. then all of these factors would be weighted and considered along with the most important factor (current battery charge left) in order to determine the current ENV. For example, assuming the above condition to be constant, then:

- If the battery level is more than 75%, the calculated ENV could be 25 – meaning that the PMP could commandeer up to a maximum of 25% of the system's resources if need be.
- If the battery level is between 51% and 75%, then the ENV could be 50 – meaning that the PMP could commandeer up to a maximum of 50% of the system's resources if need be.
- If the battery level is between 25% and 50%, then the ENV could be 75 – meaning that the PMP could commandeer up to a maximum of 75% of the system's resources if need be.
- If the battery level is less than 25%, then the ENV could be 100 – meaning that the PMP could commandeer 100% of the system's resources if need be.

However, if we alter the earlier variables such that the historical average charge was 'low' (i.e. it was only plugged in for 2 hours a day) and it regularly dropped below 25%, sources of electricity were scarce, energy expenditure was high and predicted to get even higher, etc, then the scale of the impact of the current battery level would not be as great, and the ENV would be much higher at all levels of charge (i.e. an ENV of 50 if the battery charge was less than 100%, and gradually increasing to an ENV of 100 if the battery charge dropped below 60%.

Part of the Power Management Program's job is to constantly monitor and calculate the current ENV. As a result, the current ENV could potentially change dramatically minute to minute but, in reality, the changes are much slower and much more predictable given a constant environment. However, when environments change, especially when the suit enters an environment it is not familiar with, then ENV can change dramatically quite rapidly.

The suit's current environment is very important to the Power Management Program and this is reflected in the PMP's database (a.k.a. list of *Good Stuff*) and its associated *'Learning Module'*. The database contains all the available data relating to electricity and is constantly being accessed by the Power Management Program's sensory input monitor in order to constantly be aware of what sources of electricity are currently around and how important they are.

The database consists primarily of a list of sources of electricity (i.e. electrical outlets, batteries, power lines, power generators, other electronic devices, chemical reactions, magnetic fields, etc.) along with all the data that relates to that specific source of electricity. Information in each data set relating to a specific source of electricity would include primarily information relating to the relative importance of that source of electricity (which is reflected in its *Energy Rating*) and includes data on the expected amount of energy harvested from that source, the expected energy expenditure required, etc, followed by other information associated with that source (i.e. what it looks like, where to find it, what to do to harvest/get electricity from it, etc.).

The database is *hierarchical* in nature which means that data in it is accessed in a systematic, linear way from top to bottom, based on each source's *'Energy Rating'* (ER) with higher ER data sets at the top of the list, therefore accessed first and fastest. An energy source's ER is another calculation that is made by the Power Management Program and represents the net, overall importance of that energy source. It is again based on various factors including (but not limited to):

- availability***
- actual net amount of energy acquired*****
- expected amount of net energy acquired***
- number of times successfully acquired*****
- date of last successful acquisition***
- number of times unsuccessfully acquired**
- is it an *Identified Source******, a *Possible Source****, or an *Unidentified Source***

Premade, easily accessed, low-cost, high-yield electricity sources will have a high ER while low yield, high cost, processes to possibly *make* electricity will have a much lower ER. Almost all *Identified Sources* will have a higher ER than *Possible Sources, which*, in turn, will have a higher ER than *Unidentified Sources*. Information in the database is also *fluid* which means that it constantly being modified and when data relating to a specific source of energy is changed, those changes will often be reflected in a change in that source's ER. In addition to modification of existing information[69], new data sets relating to newly discovered sources of electricity can also be created. Data is modified or added to the database by the Power Management Program's *learning module*.

This next part about the* Learning Module *and how it works is VERY IMPORTANT

----

[69] The user can also manually input information to the PMP's database.

The Learning Module:

The PMP has a '*Learning Module*' (LM) built into it as part of its basic programming. It is there so that the suits can automatically adapt themselves to ever-changing environments and thus, remain useful to the users and avoid becoming obsolete. Because the LM is part of the Power Management Program, it is also always turned on and runs automatically, independent of any user input. The LM runs according to a contingency-based adaptation model – in other words, it works using rules of **IF → THEN**[70].

The Learning Module's primary contingency rule is: "**IF** the battery level indicator increases[71] **THEN:**

1) Immediately access Memory Storage of the DIPU and playback all sensory data that was recorded *immediately preceding* the battery level indicator's increase in order to identify the source of electricity (if possible).
2) **IF** known source of energy is identified, **THEN** compare the recorded sensory information with the relevant database entries on said source of electricity and update relevant information[72] as needed.
3) **IF** no matching data is found in the existing database, **THEN** create a new, temporary data set in the "Unidentified Sources of Electricity" section of the database and input **ALL SENSORY INPUT DATA** recorded immediately preceding the identified energy surge.
4) **IF** there is more than one data set in the "Unidentified Sources of Electricity" section, **THEN** compare all sensory input data from current entry with all other data sets in this section of the database and identify similarities in sensory input data.
5) **IF** similarities are identified, **THEN** create a new data set containing all identified similarities in the "Possible Source of Electricity" section of the database.

---

[70] i.e. ***IF*** this happens, ***THEN*** do this.

[71] Which, in theory, means that there has been an influx of energy to the suit...

[72] i.e. actual net amount of energy acquired, # of times successfully acquired, date of last successful acquisition, etc.

The **Self-Preservation Program (SPP)** is the other critically important program that is built into the suit's Central Processing Unit. This program is dedicated to identifying and resolving any malfunctions with the suit. Just like the PMP, the SPP also has hardwired access to the DIPU, the ISM, as well as the CCP. However, the SPP also has much more extensive access to the suit's *Internal Systems Monitors* and monitors all of the data relating to the suit's own internal state of functioning as opposed to just the battery level because it *is dedicated to avoiding system shut-down.*

The SPP works in much the same way as the PMP does:

- It has its own database with data sets on dangers associated with system malfunction & shut-down[73] that it compares with all incoming data from the DIPU and the ISM.
- It manages and updates its database in much the same way as the PMP except that it calculates a *Relative Risk Value* (RRV) which is supposed to accurately reflect the relative risk of system shut-down associated with each danger identified in the database.
- Its ability to override and highjack the suits functions is also *progressive* and ***almost*** *absolute* (it can highjack and override **anything... except the PMP**[74]) and based on an analysis of factors related to the identified Danger which could modify the RRV (i.e. the % '*match*' of the sensory input data to the description of the danger(s) in the database, the current level of functioning, energy cost required to avoid danger/repair damage, etc.).

Because it is so important that you understand the relevance of that last point, I'm going to say it again. While the PMP and the SPP often work together without any problems, ***IF push comes to shove THEN the PMP takes precedence – which means that it will block the SPP's access to the CCP and will make the suit do whatever it needs to do to get its energy before allowing the SPP to regain access to the CCP***.

---

[73] such as 'Water', 'High Velocity Projectiles', 'Rust', 'Electrical Overload', etc.

[74] While the SPP is very important for the suit's overall functionality, it is not as important as the PMP.

In this analogy, the development of the Logic and Reason Center is when someone[75] comes along and takes ownership of the robotic power-suit so that they can use it for their purposes. This new user essentially has to install an operating system into the suit's main computer. The operating system is the program that will allow the user to control the power-suit and make it do what they want it to do. Unfortunately, the operating system is a secondary program which means that the Power Management Program and the Self-Preservation Program will continue to run in the background no matter what and, if need be, can highjack control from the user as per their programming. Understanding the interactions between the user and the power-suit is very important so I'm going to try to explain it in a little more detail.

Imagine the following situation: a guy is walking by Bestest Buy or Futurama Shop and sees the new, ultra-cool 'Titanium-Man' power-suits on sale. Being a guy, he is fascinated with all of the blinking and flashing lights and so he buys one and brings it home. On the way home, he is thinking about all of the really cool things that he is going to be able to do now with his new 'Titanium-Man' power-suit... like lift heavy things, clear out the snow from the driveway... with the flame-thrower[76], take the dog out... for a fly, mow the lawn... with its laser beams, send it to do his work while he stays home, fly to church, etc.. Luckily, the helpful sales people at the store also sold him all of the accessories he would need to have in order to make it work properly (the Operating System, the optional flame-thrower and laser-beam eye upgrades, as well as his choice of user-input devices such as a keyboard or a joystick or a mouse... or... the **SU**per **C**ontrol **K**it with **E**ye **R**ecognition – which, for a limited-time only, also includes a Bluetooth motion-activated MEGA-Control Glove!!!). Before taking his power-suit home, the techies at the store installed the operating system, all of the upgrades and ensured that the MEGA-Control Glove was properly connected to the power-suit's Central Control Panel via the operating system they installed.

---

[75] owner/user = Logic and Reason Center = Mini-U

[76] *I live in Canada... do you have any idea how cool that would be???*

Power Suits Are Fun!

So then, as soon as he gets home, he fires up the MEGA-Control Glove and immediately starts playing with his power-suit (being a guy, he never bothered to look at the instruction manual[77]). For the first couple of weeks, because he didn't read the manual, he really doesn't know what he is doing and will end up trying to make his 'Titanium-Man' power-suit do all sorts of different things – some that it was designed to be able to do, and some that it was not designed for. As he spends his days playing with (sorry... *'using'* or *'working with'...*) his new power-suit (a.k.a. toy), he notices that even though there are times when the suit responds very well to his commands, there are also a lot of times when it's really slow to respond to his commands or it does something completely different than what he told it to do and sometimes, it just doesn't respond at all.

As a result of these times when the power-suit doesn't work the way that he wants it to, he start thinking that there has to be ***something wrong*** with his 'Titanium-Man' power-suit... something must not be right in its little robotic power-suit brain... so he brings it back to the store and the techies look at it, check it out, run it through some tests and then return it to him telling him that's it's running perfectly well. So he takes it home again but then the same thing happens again! So once again, he brings it back and this time, explains in much, much, much more detail what's not working so that they can fix the problem.

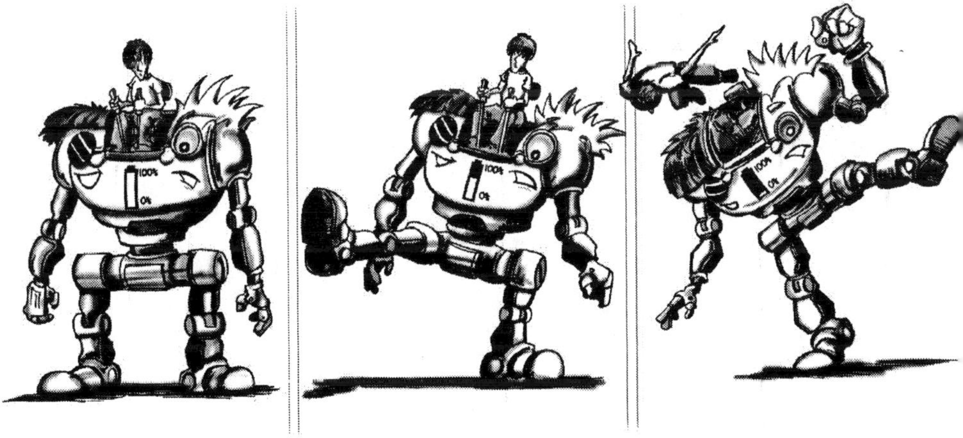

[77] Guys → It's a little booklet made of paper with writing on it that gives you instructions on how to use all of the functions built into electronic devices... seriously!

Here's the thing though... most of the time, the problem isn't with the suit... it's with the users. The problem is that they didn't read the owner's manual. It really doesn't matter why they didn't read it (i.e. they're male, it was in Chinese, it didn't come with a manual, friends told them to ignore the manual, etc.) because at the end of the day, the only way to 'fix the problem' is to understand how the power-suit works – to read about and understand the information in the Instruction Manual. If they want their Titanium-Man power-suit to work and do what they want it to do, then they need to be aware of the Power Management Program and the Self-Preservation Program and understand how those programs work and why they are there. They need to learn about and understand what's going to happen when the Titanium-Man power-suit identifies a high ENV or RRV – that the power-suit will automatically begin to commandeer more and more of the power-suit's resources/abilities/functions – which is why it will sometimes interfere with or completely block the user's ability to control it.

If the users don't read the manual and learn about how the power-suit works, then they will always be trying to find out what the problem is with their Titanium-Man power-suit (unfortunately, no refunds, no exchanges, and limited to one per person per lifetime), becoming increasingly frustrated with it over the years, constantly comparing what their power-suit can't do to what other people's power-suits can do or they might even simply give up on trying to use it at all.

IF, on the other hand, the user decides to read the instruction manual... **IF** they decide to learn about the power-suit's Power Management Program and Self-Preservation Program... **IF** they decide to research power-suits, ask people who have had suits for a long time how to use them properly... And **IF** they put this knowledge to use and start practicing how to use the power-suit properly, changing what they do by modifying when and how they use their Mega-Control-Gloves to control the power-suit **so that** the Power Management Program and Self-Preservation Program do not interfere with their control of the power-suit at an inopportune time – in the middle of lifting something really heavy... or ½ way through clearing the snow or mowing the lawn or flying the dog... or while taking a test or while giving a presentation to a large group of people or while driving or while flying overseas...

And **IF** they decide to practice making that Titanium-Man power-suit do what they want it to do... every single day... learning all of the various commands and controls and exploring/discovering what it is **really** capable of and how powerful and useful it **could** be... if it was used properly... and the user knew about all of the **potential** functions that were built in...

THEN they will really start to benefit from having that power-suit and they will stop being frustrated by it. **THEN** they will be able to do just about anything they want to do in their lives because the Titanium-Man Power-suits *really are* **incredibly powerful**... And people will look up to them and be impressed/awed by them and their power-suit ***because*** they can make their power-suit do things... things that most people have no clue how to do with *their* power-suits (because they only *skimmed through* their manual or relied on others to tell them what their suits were capable of...)... **THEN** they will have a life free of frustration and misery and limited only by their own imagination. They will be confident in their abilities, knowing that they are in control, looking back only with satisfaction at the long history of success after success after success in their lives. **THEN**, they will be happy.

Unfortunately, while it only takes a month or two to read the manual and understand the PMP and the SPP, it then takes a good 2-3 years of regular use, practicing every day, pushing it hard in order to master its control. But it is well worth it to spend the time to do so. Hard to do? Yes. Worth it? Definitely! Ask your parents or any other adult out there – what would they give for the chance to be happy all the time? To be satisfied with life? To have no regrets?

Chapter 5.89158123

And My Point Is...

To Boldly Go Where Only a Few Have Gone Before

Why would someone want to know this? Well, there are a lot of reasons why…

There's that one…

And that one…

And the other one…

Oh yeah and that one too…

And don't forget this one too!

all of which boil down to one big, all-encompassing one – for the same reason that you would want to know how to talk and read and write… except **WAY MORE HIGHER UP IMPORTANTLY THAN THOSE!!!** (*I'm serious… I'm actually not trying to be funny this time*).

That reason is that ***we are humans…***

"  !?!"

OK… well… most of us are. And humans are social creatures. Our life is made up of one social situation after another after another. Almost everything that we do in our lives involves interacting with others on some level. The social experiences in our lives are **CRITICAL** to our literal existence! (*I'm being serious again! Think about it… no socializing = no friends, no family, no lovers, no sex, no babies… = no 'Human' species anymore!!!*). Complete and total isolation from *human interaction* leads to madness, followed quickly by the disappearance of that individual's genetic existence. We exist because the humans that came before us socialized and we are genetically programmed to do the same.

When we are socializing – interacting with others – the way that we communicate with them (and the way that they communicate with us) is by saying stuff and doing stuff.

No Duh!!!

Our actions, our behaviours and our words either include us or exclude us from others. This is why what people say to us and what people do to us has such an impact on us! It's important to us! So given how much importance we, as a species, put on what people say and what people do as a method of communication, don't you think it would be very important (critical even) to be able to understand it? Interpret it? To be able to know why people around you say and do what they do? Wouldn't it be a benefit to you in your life not only to be able to accurately interpret what people are ***actually*** communicating to you but more importantly, to be able to see past that... and understand what they are ***trying*** to tell you? Wouldn't life be easier if you were able to accurately communicate back to them what ***you*** want? To know how to send the *right message* instead of Bob's or Jim's messages?[78] Wouldn't it be nice to be able to make yourself do the things that you know you should do, the things that you know will help you, the things that will make your life easier... and have it be easy to do them? Do you want to be happy? Wouldn't it be nice to be happy?

If you know this stuff, then you will know when to ignore the messages that people are sending you because they are not about something that is real... and when to ignore those same messages that Jim & Bob send to you from within. If you know this stuff and practice putting Mini-U in charge, then you will know how to change any behaviour you want to change... any behaviour that makes sense to change... which means that you would be able to change the messages that you are sending to yourself and to others around you...messages that tell everyone *who* you are. If Mini-U is in control, you can make yourself into any kind of person that you want by changing how you act – which will change how other people see you, what they know about you, what they understand about you and, as a result, how they treat you!

I don't think the real question is "why would you want to know this stuff?" but rather "How on earth can we expect people to be happy... truly happy... with no regrets at the end of their lives without knowing this stuff?!?" It's kind of like expecting a 4-year-old blind kid to hop behind the

---

[78] *Which is often useless 2-year old drivel and makes no sense and may not have anything at all to do with reality...*

wheel of his dad's truck and somehow manage to drive it from the start line five kilometres down the road to the finish line without crashing it. Seriously??? I mean, obviously, it's possible – the kid could get lucky, there may not be any cars coming down the road or any stop lights, or any trees, or any houses, or any anything (for a while anyways) but sooner or later, he's going to crash – it's not a question of **IF**, it's just a question of **WHEN**... and how serious the crashes are... and how many times he hits something on his way down the road. He *might* make it all the way to the finish line... but probably not!

"  ..."

Really?... Just ran right on over your head did she?...

"  ..."

Now why would a mother do that on purpose???

"  ..."

Well, OK, if she was a Monkey that didn't know how to drive, then it doesn't surprise me! In fact... I kind of suspected some type of serious head injury...

The sad thing is... just about every single adult out there[79] already has a bunch of 'crashes' under their belt – some worse than others. But since there is only one road ('life') and no other options available other than to keep going, after each crash, they do exactly that – they just keep on going and continue to drive like 4-year old blind kids until the next crash and then the next one and the next one after that. With each crash, their car becomes less and less and less fun to drive. And more and more of them end up badly hurt... or killed... or they simply quit and refuse to drive any

79 *Every single one that I know or have ever met... and I would be willing to bet that I could make the statement "every single adult in the world" and not be wrong...*

more... or they close their eyes and purposely aim for the cliff just wanting the nightmare to end.[80]

Happiness comes from success in life – success in finding your place in the world, success in your social life, success in achieving the goals you set, success in being able to control your actions at all times. Or in other words, happiness comes from success in getting what you want in life (good stuff) while at the same time avoiding unpleasant things (bad stuff) and doing it the right way – guided by Mini-U in accordance with his principles, values and beliefs.[81]

What I've explained so far about your brain and how it works is essentially "Life – Lesson #1: Getting to know your Brain!" It's like Driver's Ed – **Lesson #1: GETTING TO KNOW YOUR CAR – THE BRAKE THINGY, THE GAS THINGY AND EVENTUALLY, THE STEERING THINGY.**

So again, the question is why **wouldn't YOU** want to know how to drive properly so that you can get to where you want to go? And of course, don't you wish that everyone else in your life knew how to drive properly too[82]?

Are you ready for "Life – Lesson #2: Making it Work For You!"? If so, read on.

---

[80] How many times have you thought about running away somewhere far away and never coming back? About being able to just walk away and leave it all behind and never have to deal with all the stress of living? Wished you could just fall asleep and never wake up?

[81] Which is just another way of saying "in a way that's reasonable and makes sense".

[82] *I know I do... and I know that your generation should be given the chance to learn how to drive while you are still able to learn how... and before you learn all of the wrong things to do!*

Chapter 6

Are you Ready to Join

Generation 3
... or 1...
Depending on How
You Look at it?

IF you are thinking:
"I don't care... this has nothing to do with me..."

If you are completely satisfied with your life[83], then you might be right in asking that question... but then again, if you were, then why did you read up to here? The fact is, if you are going to benefit from the information that's in this book, you need to understand that what I've explained doesn't just explain some situations, sometimes. The paradigm that I have explained to you represents a completely new way of thinking, of seeing the world, and of understanding everything that people do.

If you are not convinced of the importance of understanding this, then I challenge you to put it to the test. Use it to think about and analyze people's behaviour and actively try to dissect their actions to discover which of the two drives is primarily responsible for their behaviour. Then, spend a couple of weeks thinking about and analyzing your own behaviour (especially any behaviour that you would like to change – i.e. do something you are not doing or to stop doing something you are). In order to be in control of your life, you need to activate your Mini-U, think about it and see how this all applies to your life because you need to understand what's driving a behaviour in order to have the key to changing that behaviour.

If you do not think that understanding human behaviour is important, then there has to be a reason why – some evidence that you can point to that would support your conclusion. If not...

Then ... go to Chapter 2.584592

(a.k.a Chapter 13)

(Yes... just like in a Choose-Your-Own-Adventure book!)

[83] Completely in control of your emotions and your actions, don't smoke or drink alcohol to excess, eat a healthy diet, exercise regularly, study hard, do not procrastinate, etc.

IF you are thinking:
"OK, I get it. So now what?"

Practice using your Logic and Reason Center! Train the heck out of Mini-U as often as you can, about everything you can. Practice making ***YOU (Mini-U)*** in charge of what your 'self' does and how your 'self' acts. Practice thinking about and trying to understand everyone else's behaviour in terms of Jim, Bob and Mini-U so that you can eventually start understanding your 'self' better. I'll talk about how to do this in more detail in the next couple of chapters.

Before moving on to that part of the book, I also want to briefly mention some things about people and life in general that should become obvious to you now that you know how to think about people's behaviour. This is partly to help show you how it all fits together in real life... and partly because... well... basically, there was nowhere else in the book where this stuff could go. :-D.

Every piece of advice that follows applies to most people, in most situations, most of the time. Unless you have evidence to the contrary, assume that what I am saying is true and applies to you and the people in your life.

- Humans are not creatures of logic and reason, they are creatures of emotion. DESPITE expecting everyone else to act logically and reasonably, people don't apply that same rule to themselves. Every day, they do what they do and say what they say because of their drives, NOT because they have given it thought and, after thinking about it, decided that it would be the most reasonable thing to do/say. Therefore, *you should **NOT** automatically expect that others are acting logically and reasonably because they probably aren't*. It will be much easier to understand people and their behaviour once you recognize, understand and accept that the 'reason' that they are doing something does not actually need to be a valid 'reason' – and that they might not even be able to see that it isn't a valid 'reason'.

Things to Think About...

- By default, if someone with whom you are interacting is not acting in a way that makes sense (even if they are calm), then they are being motivated by and controlled by either Jim or Bob.
- When people are 'feeling', they are not 'thinking'.
- The single most effective way to get people to do something (anything) is to find a way to entice their Jim. In other words, find a way to make it worthwhile for them to do what you want them to do. This rule also applies when it comes to making your 'self' do something too!
- Emotions are a tool that we use to communicate with others. Automatically, people will reciprocate in kind. Emotions in one person automatically evoke emotions in those around them. When the evoked emotions are a straightforward mimicry of the emotion (i.e. they are sad, so others start to feel sad, because they are sad). This is what we call 'empathy'. This is an automatic process designed to let the person who initially displayed the emotion know that their message was accepted/understood and validated and that they are part of 'the group'. The opposite is also true – if someone does not 'empathize' either in action or in words, then the message that they are sending back to the person who first displayed the emotion is that their message was not accepted/understood, was not valid and that they are being rejected from 'the group'.
- Most of the time, unless dealing with someone who is important in your life somehow, there is no real benefit to be had by pointing out more than once (i.e. arguing the point) that their actions are not 'reasonable'. *If they are over 25* and their emotions (Jim and Bob) are still louder and more in control than their Logic and Reason (Mini-U),[84] it will not matter how much evidence you try to show them, because evidence only matters to Mini-U and we already know that Mini-U is ***not*** the part of their brain that is in control of the behaviour in question. And, unfortunately, because of their age and the fact that their brain has essentially stopped developing, there is also little chance that that is going to change... **ever**!

[84] as evidenced by the fact that they are acting irrationally/unreasonably

Things to Think About...

- The word *"believe" is an emotional validation* of information – it means that the information is consistent with what's in Jim or Bob's databases. The word *"know" is an intellectual validation* of information – which means that the information is consistent with Mini-U's general database of information about the world. In other words, it represents a fact[85]. This is why people can *know* something but still find it hard to *believe* and why people can *believe* something without having any proof of it whatsoever.

- Unconditional acceptance of a person does **not** mean unconditional acceptance of their behaviour! It is very important to recognize that someone's Logic and Reason center (Mini-U) might not be in control of what they are doing at a given point in time (and depending on the person and how old they are, *"probably isn't"* would be more accurate than *"might not be"*). And if the behaviour is irrational and unreasonable, it ***should not*** be acceptable to you.

- Part of being happy is not holding onto the wrongs that other people have done to you... or to the mistakes that your Jim or Bob have made you do! Forgiving yourself and others is the only reasonable thing to do, even if you don't *feel* like you/they deserve it. If you think about it, it doesn't make sense NOT TO forgive others/yourself for the wrongs of the past. Why on earth *wouldn't* you want to purge those negative emotions? They only hurt *you*, make *you* feel crappy and *don't change/fix/undo anything*. In other words, it's a whole bunch of negative in your life for no benefit whatsoever. Forgiving someone doesn't really benefit them... it benefits YOU!

  When you truly come to understand and accept that much of what people do, and much of what you have done, was not done by choice but driven by their/your two drives and thus out of their/your control, then forgiveness of the action becomes much easier. Should you a) get mad at, and then b) stay mad at and not forgive the baby that pooped in their diapers or made a mess at the dinner table? No! It's not their fault! They couldn't help it. So what do we do? Sigh, clean up the mess and move on. And even if we do get mad at the mess, we don't

---

[85] But keep in mind that people don't always use the term 'know' properly.

stay mad at them because we know that they can't control themselves... therefore, it wasn't their fault that they did that!

- **But this does not mean that you should "Forgive and Forget!"** 'Forgive'? Yes! 'Forget'? **No**! While it makes sense to forgive, it does not make any sense at all to forget what others have done to you, *nor what Jim and Bob have made you do*. You ***need to know*** what things in your environment make your Jim and Bob react so strongly that you (mini-U) cannot override them, thus causing you to lose control over your self's behaviour. This also applies to others – you **need** to be able to recognize what it is that activates their Drives as well – so that you don't end up in the same situation as before, going through the same thing again. For example, if someone is a good friend for years, then one day, does something completely out of character for them, hurting you in the process (i.e. got drunk one night at a party you weren't at and then hit on your boyfriend/girlfriend who was at the party), does that mean that they are a bad person? That they fooled you for years, somehow hiding this side of them from you? No, it doesn't. What it means is that something happened – there was a change in their environment – that activated their Jim or Bob so much that they could not override their Drives' behavioural commands.

Should you forgive them for what they did? Yes. **BUT don't forget** what it was (the specifics of a situation) that led to that behaviour (i.e. being drunk around your boyfriend/girlfriend when you are not there) ***because*** *IF THAT SITUATION REPEATS ITSELF AGAIN, SO WILL THE BEHAVIOUR*. **It does not matter how apologetic they are or how much they assure you that they will never do it again because it was never something they decided to do in the first place!** Unless they are young (16-24) and actively trying to build up their Logic and Reason centre, then you can know for a fact that if they are in the same situation again, they will do the same thing again. They can't stop themselves. And the same applies to you too! The **ONLY** time this might not be true is if, after listening to Jim leads to a situation like this, something really-for-real bad happens to them right away because of what they did which results in that situation being put into Bob's list of things to avoid... or vice versa if it was driven by Bob initially.

<u>Things to Think About…</u>

- *The biggest 'mistakes' that people make or regrets that people have in their lives are because of broken 'trusts'.* They are the result of having trusted someone when they should not have trusted them, and, more frequently, ***they trusted themselves (their ability to override their drives) when they should not have***.

- When you have to deal with someone who is in a position of authority over you, who is doing something stupid that is negatively impacting your life (i.e a teacher who is being unfair, a parent who goes back on their word or doesn't follow through with what they said they would do, a boss who wants you to fix something that someone else screwed up, etc.), *<u>even though it's "not fair", you **should** do what you can to fix the problem</u>*. ***If*** apologizing for something that wasn't your fault will benefit you while insisting that you shouldn't have to apologize will only make the conflict continue and could cost you a job or a grade or a privilege, ***then*** it does not make sense NOT to apologize. Jim is the one saying that you shouldn't apologize because then they would win. Bob is the one who might end up making you apologize out of fear of the consequences… but if *he* is the one that makes it happen, *he* will make it happen by emotionally telling you that it ***really is*** your fault.

  Mini-U needs to take control of that situation and make you do the smart thing – apologize – for the real reason – because it is what makes sense to do – not ever *believing* that it *really-for-real* is your fault. Changing what you are doing because ***<u>Mini-U decided to</u>*** does not mean that what you were doing in the first place was wrong. It means that you are being smart – thinking rather than listening to Jim or Bob.

- If you **HAVE TO** do something (are forced to), ***<u>find a way to decide to do it yourself</u>***. Have Mini-U tell Jim that it was *your choice* to do it. Even though you know that it really-for-real wasn't, that doesn't matter since Jim doesn't care about what you know.[86] If you do this, then it won't be as bad and as negative a thing compared to if you continue to believe that you were forced into it.

---

[86] He only cares about what he senses – sees/hears/tastes/smells/feels – and telling yourself something is something he can 'hear'.

- **SLEEP!!!** – That's an instruction for success! Teenagers need about 10 hours of sleep a night. That's more than you needed when you were 12![87] Sleep is when your body does all of its important things – like grow, heal, restock energy, and move information that you learned during the day into your brain's long-term storage. Adolescence is the second most important period of growth in your life... and the last one before you get to the finished product – an adult – which is why you need lots of sleep. If you are not getting enough sleep, your body is not going to be functioning as well as it could.

  Our bodies are like cars – being awake is using it and driving it. When it comes time to do the maintenance on the car, or to modify it or pimp it out, you have to park it. You can't do those things while driving down the highway. Sleep is when we 'park' our bodies.

  One to two hours of sleep deprivation (i.e. getting only 8 or 9 hours of sleep) has a *measurable* impact on your attention, focus, memory, concentration, judgement, reaction time, emotional stability and immune functioning. The more sleep deprived you are, the bigger the negative impact. A little bit of sleep deprivation every night will end up being equivalent to a BIG problem after a while.

  What's the best thing that you can do to prevent Acne? Sleep! To get over a cold? Sleep! To help your brain learn something? Practice it... then SLEEP!!!

  What's the best way to stop feeling angry or upset? To be more in control of your emotions? Sleep! Ever notice that people's moods become progressively more extreme and unpredictable the later it gets at night (i.e. longer they go without sleep)[88]? Ever notice that no matter how bad things seem late at night, people always feel better once they have had some sleep?

  "So what!" you say... "Who cares about a little bit of learning, problems or acne... I'm having fun!" Well, think about this: a few years ago, some researchers did some experiments on sleep deprivation in

---

[87] But I'll bet that instead of moving your bedtime earlier, you are probably staying up later and getting up at the same time...

[88] It's like a computer or an x-box 360 – the longer you keep it on and play with it, the hotter it gets. If you keep going, eventually, it will overheat and shut down or simply die.

animals[89] – they artificially kept them awake with a combination of stimulants (caffeine, Red Bull, etc.) to see what the impact of prolonged sleep deprivation was on them. All along, they measured all sorts of things like their memory (how quickly they could do a maze that they knew), learning, their body's stress hormones, etc. Long story short, after an average of 6 to 7 days of sleep deprivation (no sleep at all), the rats suddenly died. No reason why – nothing detectable on autopsy or in their bloodstream that would have caused it – but their hearts just stopped suddenly, randomly, out of the blue.
After oxygen, food and water, sleep is next on the list of things that our bodies need to keep functioning.

- That screen in your head – the one you 'think' on – it's like a TV... that's broken. Because the on/off button does not work, it is on all the time. As you already know, you cannot turn it off (stop thinking about something) just because you want to. The fact is that if you do not like what's playing on the screen (the thoughts that are in your head), the only thing that you can do is change the channel (force a different thought into your mind). If Bob is holding the remote and has his channel on, switch to a channel that Jim likes[90] – repeatedly, over and over if you have to. Remember, because there can only ever be one thing on that screen at a time, changing the channel (actively choosing to think about something else) is the only way to control what's on your mind. It is hard to do at first, but it gets much easier to do as you practice doing it more and more.
- Do you have trouble falling asleep? Falling asleep is actually pretty easy if you follow these five simple steps:
    1. go somewhere quiet – no talking anywhere (including music – if it has lyrics), no random/loud noises
    2. lay down
    3. close your eyes
    4. don't move
    5. stay there, like that for 30 minutes.

---

89 *They weren't allowed to use college students as subjects any more... they tried that before and there were some really bad long-term problems that happened to the students.*
90 Jim especially likes movies, not just boring pictures.

If you can do this, I *guarantee* that you will be asleep within 30 minutes. Our brains are like computers; after 30 minutes of not being used,[91] it will automatically go into its 'screen-saver' mode (a.k.a. sleep). Thoughts running through your head do not keep you awake; it is opening your eyes and moving around trying to get comfortable that does. If thoughts and/or feelings are driving you to be uncomfortable and keeping you awake for hours, then force your brain to change the channel by actively thinking about something else – and try to maintain it for 30 minutes. That's all you have to do. Again, it sounds simple – and it is... right up to the point where you have to do it. It's actually pretty hard to do... but it is training Mini-U to over ride Jim and Bob (Bob if unpleasant thoughts and worrying are keeping you up, Jim if playing video games, chatting, texting, watching TV or doing something fun is keeping you awake).

- Do not ever underestimate the power and importance of your actions. What you ***DO*** can and will change what you think and how you feel... *regardless of the reason why you are doing it* in the first place. This is a fact, not a theory. If you act one way around one group of friends and another way around another group of friends (i.e. friends from church and friends from school), you will become the person you are acting like most of the time. You cannot maintain two opposing sets of beliefs and ways of acting for long. You will eventually adopt the one way of acting and thinking that happens most often.

- Peer pressure is more real than you think. It is hard-wired into our brains to change our 'self' to become like the people around us. If you hang out with a group of people long enough, you will start to talk, act and think like them. The more unstable you are in your feeling of belonging to your family (parents), the faster it will happen. The more time you spend around that group, the faster it will happen. It does not matter how strong you think you are, you cannot fight your biological wiring! ***The ONLY way not to succumb to peer pressure is to not be with those peers for any extended periods of time.***

[91] Not processing any information from its sensory input devices [eyes, ears, etc.] and not actively controlling your body's muscles.

Things to Think About...

- When you objectively monitor a behaviour, (keep track of and write down how much/how often you do something), it turns it into a fact. This makes it much easier to activate Mini-U's attempt to take control of that behaviour (or lack of behaviour). Keeping track of exactly how many hours of video games you play or spend chatting online or obsessing over the way your hair or your makeup or your clothes look or double/triple/quadrupple checking your work will help you to change the amount that you do that to make it more in line with what's reasonable and makes sense. *Memory* (how much you think you do it) *is not a fact and it is easily influenced and can be changed by Jim and Bob.* Don't rely on them to keep track of things you do... after all, **they can't count!!!**
- Time is the most important currency in the world. It is the only thing that everyone has only a limited amount of and once it's gone, you can never get it back. That's why people make such a big deal about time. No one wants to waste *their* time.

Chapter 7

Welcome to Driver's Ed!

Driver's Ed Rule #1: Stay Off the Sidewalk!

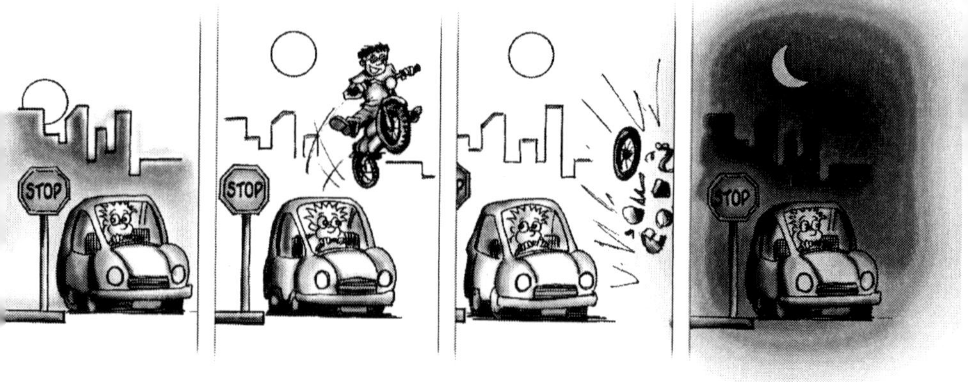

As you know, being a teenager is hard... a lot harder than it was to be a kid. The reason life suddenly got hard is because of Mini-U. With the development of Logic and Reason, suddenly (or so it seems), everything is different because you are starting to be able to see the world the way it really is... seriously! You are now finding out things that you never knew before and, sometimes, that you didn't really want to know in the first place...

"...  ?"

Yes. Exactly[92]! *(OMG... that was actually a normal question... :-0).*

One of the most important changes that take place once you become a teenager... as your understanding of the world changes... is how you see your parents, and the eventual role in your life that you will give them.

"...  ?"

NO!... I'm not talking about whether you stuff them and put them in a corner or eat them after they die.... *(I knew it was too good to be true...).*

Remember that hard-wiring I talked about earlier – the one that forced you to see your parents as perfect when you were a kid? Well, unfortunately,

---

92 That's also part of the reason why it's such a hard time for parents of adolescents as well... once you realize that they are not really "rearranging furniture" in their bedroom, they usually stop "rearranging furniture" as often.

it's still there. That urge/emotional *need* to see your parents as perfect will never go away.[93] But now, because Mini-U is working, for the first time in your life, you can have a second opinion! Now, you are able to recognize that your parents are not perfect... that they can make (and have made) lots of mistakes... that they are ***NOT really*** the perfect people you thought they were. Suddenly, you can see them for who they truly are – be that good, bad, or otherwise[94].

Do you remember how you felt when you found out/figured out the truth about Santa? That feeling of sadness and loss? The hurt? (This is what it's like for most kids. But for some who have really big, sensitive Bobs[95], it's actually a relief – cuz sometimes, they are *terrified* of Santa – because he's creepy... always watching you... when you're sleeping... when you're awake... sneaking into your home without you ever seeing him... bypassing all security.). Well, suddenly realizing that your parents aren't perfect is nothing like that. Finding out about Santa is like stubbing your toe while, for a lot of teenagers, figuring out the truth about their parents is like slowly cutting off their leg with a butter knife over the course of a couple of years... except that most teenagers never feel any of this.

Instead, most of the time, those feeling of pain and loss and insecurity that come from Bob are masked by Jim's anger – hot, raging, intense anger! Have you ever noticed that your parents have the capacity to bring out the most intense anger in you? That you can become angrier with them than you have ever been in your life... at anyone!

---

[93] Regardless of the kinds of parents that you have, throughout your life, you will most likely find yourself repeatedly turning to them for help, advice, rescue, etc. Emotionally, you will always *believe* that parents are perfect... even once you *know* that they are not. It will almost always feel wrong to think negatively about your parents and will often lead to feeling guilty for doing it. How much guilt and negative emotion is evoked depends on how loud your Bob is compared to your Jim.

[94] like realizing that they are *only* highly intelligent monkeys ☺

[95] *ROTFLMAO... OMG.... Apparently I, my spellchecker, and a couple of others missed a really bad typo in that last sentence... "Bobs" had an extra O... Thanks to LD for catching that :).*

Is it hard to understand why? Not really... after all, how could they say/do that to you!!! They are so... ***UNFAIR!!!***[96] Now that you are older, you understand what it means when they criticize you... and it burns into your soul... and it makes you even angrier! You feel betrayed by the ones you trusted the most... often feeling like they have been lying to you all this time.

Most of the time, these feelings are subconscious and we aren't even aware of them being there... except when they bubble over every now and then. Now, how angry you get and how guilty you feel depend on the following:

1. How loud are your Bob [louder = more guilty feelings] and your Jim [louder = more angry feelings].
2. How close to really-for-real "perfect" are your parents? [The further they are from being really-for-real perfect, the more intense and longer-lasting the feelings of anger and guilt will be.]

Can you see the problem yet? Unfortunately, this anger and rage is directed at your **parents** – *the only people in the world who are biologically protected against you having those kinds of feelings towards them*. This is often why, once the anger fades, it is replaced by guilt.[97] And then, a funny thing happens – you forget about what happened to make you so angry and you go back to being the kid who loves their wonderful parents until the next time they do something like that again... and again... and again... and again.

Most people spend their teen years going back and forth between feeling angry and hating their parents to feeling guilty for hating them to loving them and wanting to have unconditional acceptance from them and approval of everything they do and all the choices they make, to be valued so much by their parents that they would do anything, give them anything... which never happens. Nor should it since it would not make

---

[96] or whatever other colourful adjectives you tend to use.

[97] Bob: "What's wrong with you that you would dare think something like that about your parents... they are ***Mom*** and ***Dad***!!! → Cut #1 with a butter knife.

any sense for parents to do that[98]... but neither Jim nor Bob really care whether or not it's a good thing to want... they *both* want it! There are already too many adults in the world already who cannot escape that cycle – who continue to go back to their parents only to get emotionally cut again and again – for as long as their parents are alive. In fact, many parents are still stuck in that cycle with their own parents – have you ever been forced to go see grandparents who are mean, cranky and just not nice? Does it make sense for a parent to make a child interact with someone like that???

Now, some teenagers out there will have gotten lucky and were born to people who are very good parents. For them, that period of emotional transition doesn't last very long and is pretty easy to handle.[99]

For most people however, their parents are average parents – which means that it will likely be a tough transition for them. For most teenagers, fifteen to seventeen are the roughest years and are usually filled with a lot of conflict, anger and fighting with their parents. But by the time they are eighteen or nineteen, the fighting will usually have settled down quite a bit. Don't get me wrong, there will still be some arguments and fights (over and over and over for many years still) around issues like 'trust', their 'life choices', their 'screw-ups', etc. but despite the ongoing conflict, the urge to please their parents, *wanting* their approval... that will continue on, and on, and on, and on,.... for a very long time.

Now, unfortunately, some people... some of you reading this right now... got totally screwed and ended up being born to people who were either not ready to be, or were simply *unable*[100] to be, good parents. They were ***limited*** in what they could do and what type of parent they could be right

---

[98] Remember, unconditional acceptance of a person does **not** mean unconditional acceptance of their behaviour! It is the same distinction as I suggest you make with yourself – hate your Bob or Jim for what they make you to do... but don't hate yourself for it.

[99] How do you know if this is you? Well, if/when you're 16 or older, then, the majority of the time, you still like being at home, still like your parents, trust their advice and don't often get angry or fight with them anymore.

[100] for any number of reasons, and believe me, there are a TON of reasons that people simply **cannot** be 'good' parents which include having a mental illness, having substance abuse problems, having other physical or emotional limitations and, most commonly, they were ***never taught how to be one!***

from the start. Teenagers who have limited parents are still getting angry at their parents and/or feeling guilty about stuff that's going on between them just like teenagers who have 'average' parents – except that the conflict and fighting will be happening **a lot more often and is a lot more intense**. If you are one of those teenagers unlucky enough to belong to this group, your life probably 'sucks' right now... and you are probably not happy **most** of the time.

Teenagers who have limited parents have often wanted and wished for a different life... but don't really know what they want their life to be like... except to know for sure that they sure as hell do not want the one they have.

The fact of the matter is though, that I ***know*** (even if you don't) that ***it*** (getting shafted as far as parents go) is *completely and entirely* the reason that you are where you are in your life right now! It is the reason why you feel the way you feel and the reason why you are not happy.[101] Believe me, ... I wish that there was some way to undo your past... right the wrongs... give you a different life... but there isn't. BUT, that doesn't mean that it's hopeless and that you can't end up becoming happy and living a satisfying, fulfilling life. *You can still change your life... if you want to*.

Yes, it is your parents' choices and behaviours (how they raised you and what they taught you) that have made your life what it is as of today. But once you read this book, ... once you *know* what to do... where your life goes and the kind of person that you end up becoming... that's going to depend COMPLETELY on you – your choices and your actions – from here on out! You can change your life to make it into what you want it to be. It's not easy, but it's easily worth it!

---

[101] *Back to the Driving analogy with Parents = First Driving Instructor. But unfortunately, anyone who wants to can become a Driving Instructor [parent]. Anyone can sign up and take on a student driver [baby/child] and try to teach them everything that they know about Driving... or don't know... or think they know but don't really. Good First Driving Instructor = Good Driving Skills = less accidents... but a crappy First Driving Instructor = Crappy Driver = Demolition Derby.*

Driver's Ed Rule #1: Stay Off the Sidewalk!

Now, some of you may have tried to change your lives before but unfortunately, unless you know ***what you need to do*** to change things, you can put in a lot of time and energy and effort without seeing much success. It's like that door at the mall that you try to push open... unless you realize that you have to ***pull*** on it instead of pushing it, you will end up tired and exhausted, getting nowhere...

Not that I've ever done THAT...... :-S

And then, after putting in all that effort and work, when you go nowhere, you eventually end up getting discouraged and giving up... believing that it simply cannot be done. I'm here to tell you that that's not true! It can be done... you just need to know how to do it.

Knowing what to do and how to do it is the most important step in starting to change your life.

It's the reason that I wrote this book. The real value of the information you've read so far is that once you know why people do the things that they do, and more importantly, ***why you do the things that you do*** – once you understand the *"why?"* – then you can change that behaviour **by changing the *"why"***. *That's really what this book is all about – explaining to you how to change your life so that, if you ever want to, you can.*

If you fall into the group of teenagers who have limited parents, please make sure that you read Chapter 10 carefully. After the first couple of chapters in this book, it is **the most important chapter for you to read**! Unfortunately, if you fall into this group, you will need to be able to understand your parents and their behaviour and learn to think of them in a very specific way in order to be able to make use of anything else that's in this book.

The following three chapters are not meant to be read by everyone!!!

Chapter 8 is for those of you who have average parents (which is what most of you reading this will have). Chapter 9 is for those of you who have good parents. Chapter 10 is for those of you with ***limited*** parents – limited in how well they understand children's needs and limited in their ability to act appropriately. Limited because of their intellectual deficiencies, emotional problems, physical limitations, mental health issues, substance abuse issues, or, for whatever other reasons, fall into the category of TFUP.[102]

You need to think about and decide which of the following three chapters to read (8, 9, or 10) before moving on to chapter 11.

"...  ?"

YES... YOU!!!

"?"

And you too.

"...  ?"

NO!!! You can't just read the one she reads... YOU need to decide, for yourself, which one applies to YOUR parents.

"...  ?"

---

[102] *It's a diagnostic acronym - like FUBAR.*

… … … no… … … there is no chapter for parents who are sophisticated, highly intelligent monkeys… that's going to be in the next book, right after the chapter on understanding parents who are eggplants!

"… ?"

… … … tomorrow… only available in Siberia… in person… for a limited time… Hurry!!!

Chapter 8

Understanding "Average", Everyday, Pretty Normal Parents

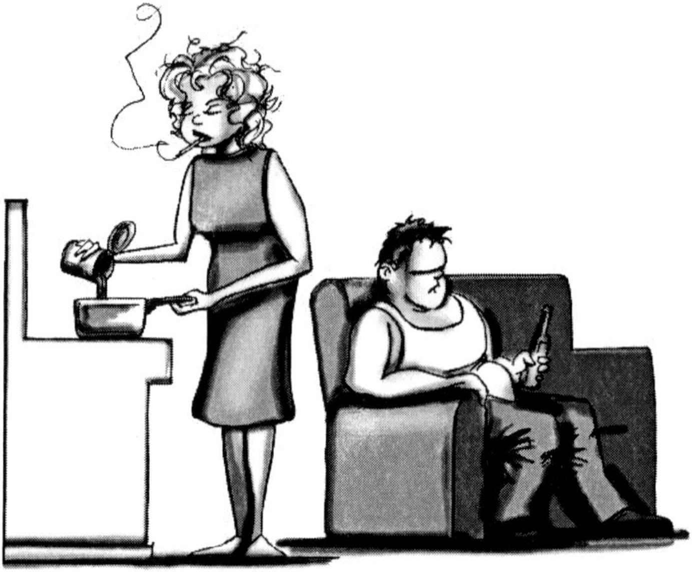

If you have "Average" Parents...

Understanding your parents is about recognizing what's really-for-real real and true about them – as people, and as parents. If you're at least sixteen years old, then you have undoubtedly figured out that your parents are not the "perfect" people that you once thought they were (in fact, you might not even remember **ever** thinking that they were perfect). By now, you can see that they are just average, every-day human beings – sometimes wrong in what they say, sometimes unfair in how they treat you or others, sometimes hypocritical – telling you to do something that they themselves do not do or telling you not to do something that they are doing themselves.

The simple fact is that they, like most people out there, have a Logic and Reason Centre with a *volume* somewhere around 5... which means that they are sometimes not listening to Logic and Reason (or are simply unable to because their Drives are too loud) and are therefore acting completely and totally irrationally. In other words, they will sometimes lose their temper and end up saying and doing things that they *know* are stupid. They will sometimes get really anxious and, as a result of being unable to control their own anxiety and what it makes them do, be completely over-protective and set ridiculous limits on what you are allowed to do, or who you are allowed to see or talk to. They will try to, single-handedly, protect you from whatever bad thing in the world it is that they are worried about by essentially not letting you anywhere near it.

Unfortunately, prior to Mini-U joining the game, you thought they were perfect. Now, you "suddenly realize what they are really like"[103] – which sucks... big time. This 'sudden' realization automatically leads to feelings of disappointment and anger, feelings of betrayal, feelings of isolation and loneliness and feeling 'lost'. For some teenagers, there is some conscious awareness of these feelings; they can tell that something emotionally powerful is there, simmering just beneath the surface. However, most teenagers aren't consciously aware of those feelings... until something happens to cause them to boil over and explode. That 'something' is usually something small, often insignificant... except for the 'theme' that the event represents. When this emotional explosion happens, the intensity of those emotions is far above and beyond what would be considered a "normal" emotional reaction to that situation – because of the subconscious build-up of all of that negative emotional pressure that developed because of Mini-U's developing awareness of reality.

When teenagers' awareness of the world and of their parents changes, they often start questioning everything they thought they knew about everything. After all, if they were **THAT** wrong about their parents, then what else were they wrong about? And if they no longer admire their parents and stop wanting to be like them when they grow up, then they now have to figure out who they **DO** want to be like. When teenagers no longer want to be part of their parents' 'herd', they start to feel lonely and isolated, feeling like they don't belong anywhere. It's these feelings that often drive teenagers to desperately start looking for a new 'herd' – a group of people that will accept them and understand them – unlike their parents. It is this feeling of no longer belonging to their parents' 'herd' – the sense of no longer believing what their parents believe and no longer wanting to be like their parents that drives most teenagers to suddenly

[103] *quoted directly from a patient of mine who was 14 at the time*

start changing who they are – what they look like and how they act – and experimenting (to see if this group is the one they want to belong to)[104].

So then, given that you now know what happens to most teenagers at an emotional level and why it happens, is there anything that you can do to avoid it? Do you want to avoid it? **SHOULD** you avoid it? Yes! I don't know... and yeah, it makes sense to avoid it if you can.

"...  ?"

Didn't you leave yet?

"...  !"

Siberia!!! Google it!

"...  !!!"

OMG.... NOT CYBERIA.... S-I-B-E-R-I-A!!! Now GO!!!! HURRY!!!!!

I'm so sorry that he's part of your generation... I think that he single-handedly dropped the average IQ in this room by a good 30 points!

OK, back to the question. How can you avoid that emotional disaster (or fix it if you're already in the middle of it)? What do you need to know about your parents that will help make those feelings less intense, and eventually go away? What do you need to *understand* about them? Well, the answer to that question is actually pretty simple... simple in theory, but difficult in practice. What teenagers and young adults need to do in order to escape those feelings we just talked about is to ***build an understanding of their parents using Mini-U instead of Bob AND/OR Jim.*** However, this is much easier said than done because Bob and Jim are going to be trying to

---

[104] It's what their parents and other adults in their lives call 'being rebellious'

influence them every step of the way. They will be putting thoughts into their head and answering the questions they ask themselves as they try to figure it all out.

?"

YES!!! Exactly like the guy who just left! Except that because the statements that they make come from within their own heads, it makes it much harder to recognize that it's Jim or Bob talking. In fact, the only reliable way to tell is to double check every thought, every statement, and every conclusion that comes into your mind with your 'Dummy Detector' – Mini-U! In other words, you have to check and see if they ***make sense.*** The best way to do that is to say it (the thought or conclusion) to yourself, or to others, out loud. When you say something out loud, you force it to be processed through Mini-U. Have you ever had an idea or thought something that *you thought* made sense... right up until you said it out loud (usually when trying to explain it to someone else) and only then did you realize that it didn't really make sense?[105] Or what about when you or someone you know says something, believing that it's a fact (based on reality) but when questioned about it says that "It's really hard to explain..." and so they don't explain it... because they can't? These are all situations where Jim or Bob have 'told' us something and followed it up by assuring us that it's true and it makes sense... even though it doesn't but we accept it as true because we trust them. **DON'T TRUST THEM!!!** Force yourself to give yourself the evidence behind every conclusion that comes into your head. It's the only sure way of knowing that you're not making a mistake.

When teenagers are able to do this, they come to some general conclusions about their parents that help defuse those negative emotions. I could tell you what they are... but it's always best if you figure it out yourself. Nothing that anyone tells you is ever going to be as powerful as if you came to that conclusion because you figured it out yourself. So I'm going to suggest that you stop reading here. Go and think about it. Try to solve the problem on your own. Think about your parents and try and

---

[105] Ever heard someone say "That made a lot more sense in my head!"?

figure out what would be really important to know about them and who they are. Think of a recent fight that you had with them and see if you can understand what the fight was about, why they did what they did and said what they said. Say it out loud. Write it out. Then when you've done that come back here and keep reading and check your answers against the ones in this book.[106]

Or, if you prefer, you can just keep on reading to find out the answers from me. If you do decide to do that, you should still go back afterwards and confirm it for yourself.

These are the answers/understandings you should have come up with.

Your parents are only human – they make mistakes, have made mistakes and will make many, many more mistakes over the years. The most important thing for your Mini-U to understand about them is that they only have a Mini-U (Logic and Reason Centre) with a volume of around 5 or 6 while their Bob (Harm Avoidance Drive) and their Jim (Pleasure Seeking Drive) are capable of volumes of 10 – just like everybody else. Now, once you understand this and accept it, you will see that what it means is:

A LOT of the bad stuff that you have experienced from them in the past – and will continue to experience from them – is not really under their control; it happened and will keep happening because either their Jim or Bob is in control of their behaviour a lot of the time… which also means that *there probably isn't any* **REAL**, *valid "reason" for those behaviours.*

So how do you know which pieces of information coming from them to take seriously? How can you tell what's relevant to your life, for real? How can you tell ***when*** to actually listen to them and ***when*** to actively think about what they say and do, and then filter out and ignore the

---

106 Just like you should do with Math homework – flipping to the back of the textbook and copying down the answers to the questions doesn't really help you understand it… but doing it and then checking the answers and, most importantly, when what you came up with is different than what's at the back of the book, figuring out *why* your answers don't match is the important part.

crap[107]? Well, it's actually quite simple; you need to start thinking about what they say and actively filtering whenever there is a lot of emotion present when they are saying/doing whatever it is that they are saying/doing.

And, fortunately, because you have typical, average, pretty normal parents, you might even be able to use them as a resource. Chances are that if you ask them later, **when they are calm** and not emotional, about what they **really** *think* about what they said or did when they were angry or upset, then they will probably tell you what they *really* think. Do they *really* think that you are a total screw-up? Do they *really* think that you will never make anything of yourself? Do they *really* think that you can't get anything right? Do they *really* think that it was fair to ground you for a year? Did they *really* mean it when they called you a "______"? Granted, sometimes, you still won't get a *real* answer because they might become defensive right away (unfortunately, most adults in the world have a very hard time admitting that they made a mistake and instead try to justify their actions through the use of flawed logic). But if you try asking them in this way, at least you have a chance of getting a '*real*' answer.

Now, if you can't get a *real* answer from them, or your own Bob won't let you bring it up with them, that's OK because there is another easy way to figure it out – *ask yourself* – **when YOU are not in an emotional state – AND/OR** *ask a friend* or another adult that you trust, if what they said/did made sense given what was going on at the time. When you are trying to figure it out yourself, the first thing to do is to dissect the event in as much detail as you can (details help to keep it objective – based on facts) and then, when you consider all of the facts – what you know is true and real – ask yourself/friend/other adult if what they said or did was reasonable. If the answer to that question is "No!" then the next step is to ask yourself/friend/other adult what would have been a reasonable thing to have said/done given the facts of the situation – because that's what *should* have happened.

---

[107] because either their Jim or Bob is in control

Now, when you are asking yourself/friend/other adult these questions and coming up with answers, there are some simple 'clues' that can help guide you. The first clue to use when analyzing statements that they make is to go over exactly what they said, word-for-word. If they used the terms "always" or "never", 99% of the time, you can stop right there. You see, there is a huge difference between the descriptive terms "always" and "never" (which are almost exclusively used by Jim and Bob[108]) and the terms "sometimes", "occasionally", "rarely", or "frequently" (which is Mini-U's language[109]).

The second clue to look for is the presence of emotion at the time of the event. It's pretty easy to tell if they are feeling angry or irritated (Jim), but what about if they're feeling anxious? Or scared? Or mildly uncomfortable? Those emotions tend to be much harder to identify in parents and unfortunately, anxiety-driven (Bob-controlled) behaviour is common, but not as common as Jim-driven behaviour, for most parents. In general, if you think about the situation and the behavioural outcome was not a logical one, and you're pretty sure that they weren't "angry" at you, then it's highly likely that there was some degree of anxiety present influencing their behaviour. In general, moms are more likely than dads to have anxiety and both parents are more likely to have anxiety present when dealing with daughters than with sons.

You should also be aware that there are some parents who have a lot of anxiety, and it's often the only emotion present and unfortunately, it's present almost all the time. So how can you tell if one or both of your parents fit into this category? Well, generally speaking, by the time you're old enough to be reading this book, you should also be able to think about and identify (roughly) the relative volumes of your parents' Jims and Bobs. By now, you know your parents well enough to be able to identify if they are worriers or not, if they get stressed easily or not, if they are control freaks or not, if they are pessimists or not, if they focus only on the negative, and spend most of their time pointing out what could be better, if it seems like they aren't satisfied by anything, if they seem to always

---

108 *Remember... Jim and Bob are dumb as stumps and can't count* ☹

109 *Because he knows how to count!* ☺

have something to complain about, if they are clean freaks, etc. Parents with overly-loud Bobs (a.k.a. *worriers*) are almost always in a state of worry about something or other and only sometimes, recognize that worrying as irrational. What this means for you is that, if one of your parents is a worrier, you should, *always* double check with your own brain (i.e. ask Mini-U) to figure out if something they are saying or doing makes any sense or not.

****WARNING****

When you are thinking about what your parents are doing or saying, **DON'T then tell them that they are not making any sense** – that will only make the situation worse! Keep in mind that in the middle of the situation, they are not thinking rationally so to try to point that out isn't going to make any difference at all. If your Jim is pushing you, forcing you to say something, then **ONLY** ask them to explain to you how they came to that conclusion. You can say that as a way of trying to, in a roundabout way, encourage them into using their Logic and Reason Centre - if you must - but understand that *the most likely outcome of any type of challenge to what they are saying is not going to be a good one for you.* So, given that you now know this, does it really make sense to say something to them if it's not going to help change them and it's only going to hurt you???

Understanding your parents is not about blaming them for the mistakes and screw-ups that they have made. And it's not about figuring them out so that you can show them how to change what they are doing because they can't. Rather, it is about recognizing that the lower volume of their Logic and Reason Center limits the usefulness of the information that they give you. And that a lot of the information/feedback that they give you (in terms of what they say and what they do) may simply need to be put aside as being useless, meaningless and false[110].

The goal of understanding your parents is to be able to take the positive interactions and memories that come from them and leave the negative ones behind – by minimizing/eliminating the impact of those negative

[110] But not in a confrontational way!

ones by actively filtering them out of your head as soon as you recognize them as not being true.

Always remember that the negative interactions that come from them – that false, useless, grossly exaggerated information – is not coming from them! It's coming from their 2 drives (Jim & Bob) and even though they don't really mean it, they can't help it and can't stop doing it either because they aren't in control of their Jim and Bob any more than you are.

When it comes to your parents, it is important for you to understand that, unfortunately, they will **always** be the way they are – with a louder Jim and Bob than Mini-U and as such, often not in control of their behaviour. Here's the good news though. The difference between you and them is that, if you decide to work out your Mini-U daily, in a year or two, you (Mini-U) will be in control of your behaviour rather than blindly following Jim and Bob's orders. Which means that you will not be making a lot of mistakes in your life... which means that you will be able to enjoy life a lot more... which is a critically important part of being happy. In other words, there's still hope for you!

Chapter 9

Understanding “Good” Parents

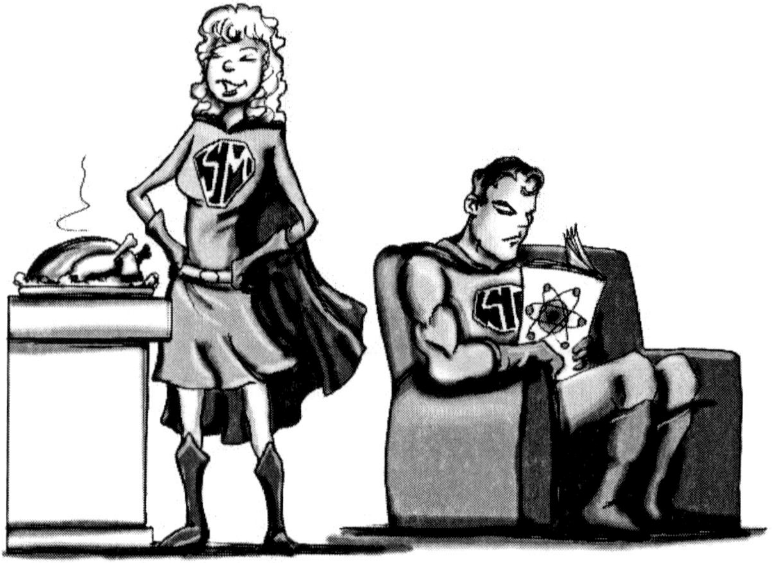

<u>If you have "Good" Parents...</u>

Congratulations! You got lucky. Not much for you to do other than fine tune those little things. For you, the biggest challenge that you are going to have is trying to figure out what you want to do with your life (school, job, etc.). The biggest urge/drive that you are going to have is to follow in your parents' footsteps. The challenge/difficulty that you might have is going to be dealing with your Bob if you happen to want to do something else with your life.

If you happen to want to be something that your parents do not strongly approve of, Bob will not like that. In Bob's view, because your parents are good, than being 'them' is being 'good'. To be something that is **not** 'them' is **not** 'good' and "not good" is ***bad***. In other words, you will feel guilty and uncomfortable with the idea of 'not wanting to be just like your parents' – even though it isn't wrong to do so[111]. Having said that, if you've taken the time to build up Mini-U, then dealing with those feelings shouldn't be too difficult a task and Bob shouldn't stop you.

---

[111] *Desiree, Celeste, Connlan - this does not apply to you!!! You'll all be in serious trouble if you don't go to medical school like me!*

Chapter 10

Understanding "Bad", Limited, TFU Parents

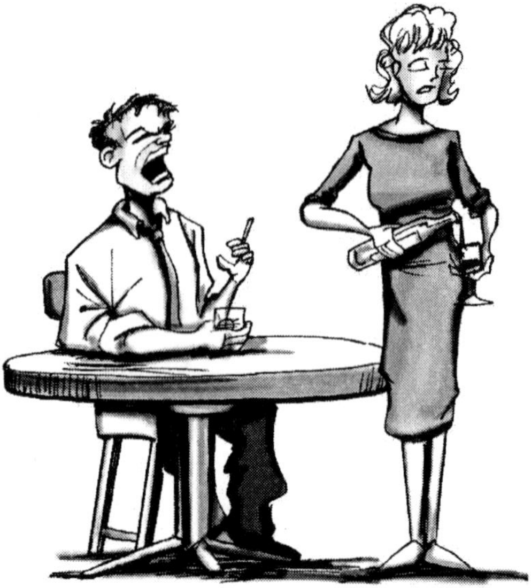

If you have 'Limited' parents...

As you already know, it sucks being you... and it has sucked being you for a long time (about 15-16 years or so...). I'm sorry that you were unlucky in terms of who your parents are. I want you to know that no matter what you have been through and no matter where you are right now, things can change. Your life can become better and you can learn to be happy just as easily as anyone else. I want you to know that you guys are the main reason that I wrote this book – you guys are *my* inspiration.

Every day, in my office, I see teenagers who have such amazing potential – intelligent, beautiful, creative, talented, friendly, funny... – but who can't see it themselves. Who can't bring themselves to believe that they are worthwhile and have value as an individual. Who are depressed and sad and lonely because they believe that they are unlovable, that they will never fit in anywhere, that there is something so fundamentally wrong with them that they sometimes wonder why they even bother waking up in the mornings. Who are angry at their parents, at their teachers, at the world because *it's not fair*... angry because they don't fit in and they are past the point of being sad about it and have become mad about it. Who want to hurt others so that others will know how they feel... and maybe then, the hurting will stop...

Every day, I see teenagers who come from TFUPs change and grow and stop hurting and start being happy, start being in control of their lives, start believing that they are worthwhile, start feeling good about themselves and who they are, and start seeing a possibility for a happy future for themselves. And all it took for them to get there was for someone to explain it[112] to them (over and over, mind you, but that's not a surprise since we're trying to undo 15 years of learning and re-train the brain to think differently). And because I have seen so much good come out of teenagers who, according to other people, would never amount to much or were beyond help, I couldn't justify not taking the time to write this book.

So then, what do you guys need to know? Well, for starters, where you are right now, how you feel about yourself and your life, how happy you are → it's not your fault that you are there. It's theirs... no matter what they say. Now, to be clear, when I say "fault", I mean that their actions are the reason that you are where you are right now. Yes, your actions may have contributed to you ending up where you are, but your actions are and have been controlled by the people around you and your environment for pretty much all of your life so far. *If your parents had done things differently[113], you would not be where you are today*. Your life would be completely different.

If you want to change your life to be something different than what it is right now, then the first step to doing that is to understand and accept this as fact... because it is. You need to understand this basic premise because you need to know how to explain ***to yourself*** **WHY** you do the things that you do from here on out – so that you can change what you ***do*** – and make

---

[112] what they needed to know about their thoughts, their emotions, their behaviour and their parents

[113] had changed how they acted around you, changed what they said to you when you were growing up, modified the stuff that you were exposed to, treated you appropriately based on your personality and temperament, and taught you what you needed to know as a child

your life become what **YOU** want it to be! If you are not happy, if your life is not what you want it to be, you need to believe and to ***know*** that it's fixable! ***I know it's fixable but YOU are the one that needs to know it!***

You can find happiness and be at peace in your life! I promise you that if you read this book, work at understanding it and start *doing the things that you need to do* in order to fix your 'life', it can and will get better. **It will take time – 2-3 years of hard work or 4-5 years of not-so-hard work** – but if you start now[114], you **can** fix it!

A couple of quick things about your past that, if it applies to you, you also need to know now[115]:

If you were "diagnosed" with some sort of mental illness or psychiatric problem as a child, it *might* not really be there.

- **If** you were diagnosed with "**Bipolar Disorder**" or told you were "Bipolar" **prior to the age of 12 → IT'S NOT TRUE!!!** You don't have Bipolar Disorder! Yes, your moods are probably all over the place and they go up and down to extremes like a yoyo – but it's not because you have Bipolar Disorder – it's probably because of the way you were raised. This is called mood *hyper-reactivity*... and we're all born that way to begin with. It's the way a 3 year old deals with life – extreme emotional reactions up and down. If you still experience this it's because you haven't learned how to control your emotions yet. That's all. The good news is that you *can learn to regulate your emotions.*

  It doesn't matter if your parents have "Bipolar Disorder" too – all that means is that you are at an increased risk of developing Bipolar Disorder in your life – it does NOT mean that you have it too – even if the way you act and the way that your moods look are an awful lot like those of your "Bipolar" parent(s). Remember – you learn what

[114] I am assuming that you are somewhere between the ages of 16 and 19

[115] JIC you don't read to the end of the chapter...

they teach – through their actions and your observations of their actions – and are hard-wired to try to become exactly like them… so should it be any wonder that you might act a lot like they do?

- If you were diagnosed with **ADHD** → Maybe it's true, maybe not. Don't assume you have it… and *don't* assume you don't. *You need to find out if you do.* ADHD is a ***very*** genetic illness. If one of your parents has ADHD, there is about a 70% chance you will too. Keep in mind that they might not even know they have it or they might be in denial about it so asking them might not be of any benefit. Unlike other Mental Illnesses (like Bipolar Disorder), you don't develop it later in life – you will have had it all your life. It really shouldn't be diagnosed in kids until about 7 or 8 since before that age, a child's normal brain immaturity mimics its symptoms – but if it's there, then the 'wiring problem' has been there all along.

ATTENTION-DEFICIT HYPERACTIVITY DISORDER (ADHD) IS SOMETHING THAT CAUSES A LOT OF PROBLEMS IN PEOPLES' LIVES – IT MAKES THEIR LIVES A LOT HARDER[116]

BUT IT CAN BE VERY EASILY TREATED

WHICH WILL MAKE LIFE MUCH EASIER!

You are old enough now to be reliable when it comes to reporting to the doctor what symptoms of ADHD you have, if any. BUT… keep in mind that if you have ADHD, you are NOT the best person to tell if it is there or not, because you will have been like that your entire life, so you won't know any other way of thinking or acting… besides which – you have to be able to pay attention to stuff going on around you and your reactions to them in order to be able to notice if you are or are not missing things (because you weren't paying attention). And if you have Attention-Deficit Hyperactivity Disorder, it's hard for you to pay attention… and so you likely have never noticed that you aren't paying attention! Once again, you have to rely on other people's perspectives – what do other people say? (Ask them if you don't know).

[116] compared to people without ADHD

- If you were diagnosed with **Oppositional Defiant Disorder (ODD)** or **Conduct Disorder (CD)** → it's probably accurate... but the thing is, those diagnoses are not really '*Mental Illnesses*' like schizophrenia or Bipolar Disorder or ADHD... they are labels that describe clusters of specific behaviours that kids can exhibit. Now, if you had seriously messed up parents, I would totally expect that you would act like that; in fact, I would be surprised if you didn't have 'bad behaviour' as a child. Keep in mind that, once again, kids do what they see parents do and act like their parents act (and have the same genetic 'Temperament' [relative volume of Jim vs. Bob] as their parents). So if your parents have a very quiet Bob, therefore, a very loud Jim by comparison, it's very likely that you do too! And if their behaviour is not good... inappropriate... basically totally messed up (which is a given if you are reading this chapter) – then unfortunately, the only role models you have ever had, and the only lessons you have ever learned about how to behave, are also 'messed up'. You have undoubtedly learned some pretty crappy behaviours and are 'limited' in your own knowledge of appropriate ways to interact with other people. Fortunately, you can fix that... you can learn better ways of behaving and interacting with others... you can learn to be in control of Jim rather than letting him mess up your life... **but ONLY if you want to**.

Now that I have that out of the way, back to explaining your parents to you. What is a 'limited' parent? These are parents that are very often wrong in their interpretation of the world around them and subsequently, in their reactions to things. These are parents that are very hurtful, mean, unfair and inappropriate in the things that they have said and done to you and others throughout your life. The term '*Limited*' refers to the fact that they are ***limited in their ability to control their behaviour***. In other words, the main problem that 'Limited' parents have is that their Mini-U (Logic and Reason) isn't very loud at all – usually about a 3 or a 4... and in some cases, far, far quieter still.

What this means is that most of the time, Jim and/or Bob are in control of their behaviour (what they say and what they do) and as a result, they will almost always act without ever *thinking about what they are doing*. In other words, they lose their temper all the time and often say and do things that are stupid.[117] They might have a ton of anxiety themselves and, because they are unable to control it, become completely over-protective or set ridiculous limits on what you are allowed to do, who you are allowed to see, talk to, etc.. In essence, for most of your life, they have been completely unable to provide you with a good, appropriate behavioural role model for you to see, learn from, and imitate.

Because you have 'Limited' parents, you have undoubtedly already figured out by now that they are **NOT** the 'perfect' people that you once thought they were when you were a kid. What teenagers tend to notice first about 'Limited' parents is that they are very hypocritical – telling you to do/not to do something that they themselves do not do/do. Unfortunately, prior to Mini-U joining the game, you thought they were awesome parents, but now, you "suddenly realize what they are really like"[118] – which sucks big time given how far (*so very, very, very far*...) they are from that 'perfect' image you had of them in your brain while you were growing up.

What happens next, after a teenager comes to this realization, is very predictable; every teenager who grew up in a home with 'Limited' parents has the same basic emotional reaction to this information - disappointment, loss (sadness), betrayal, isolation (feeling like you don't belong there any more), and anger (*usually, a hell of a lot of it*). If you have a loud Jim, then the emotion you will be most aware of is the intense anger. If you have a loud Bob, the feeling you will be most aware of are the sadness, isolation and overall feeling of emptiness, as well as guilt (for being angry [consciously or subconsciously] at them).

For some teenagers, there is some awareness of these emotions (usually the anger) always simmering, just beneath the surface, making you constantly feel like something just isn't right – unhappy, uneasy,

---

[117] They might or might not *know* that it's stupid...

[118] *Quoted directly from a patient of mine who was 14 at the time*

uncomfortable, irritated and grouchy. And this muddle of feelings that they often can't identify just continues, day in and day out, often bubbling over and spilling out into their every-day life, triggered by the smallest things, every-day things like not catching the green light and being stuck at the red... or someone not calling them right when they said they would... or people being late for something and them having to wait... or any other tiny little thing that really doesn't matter. And when that happens, they often feel intense negative emotions (despair, rage, etc.) that are far more intense than what they would expect based on what's actually going on in their life.

In general, what teenagers notice most (if they are able to take a step back and observe their own behaviour) is that their emotional reactions to every-day life are all far above and beyond what would be considered a "normal" emotional reaction to that situation (especially the anger). The reason for this? Well, it's because of their 'Limited' parents – because of the build-up of all of that negative emotional pressure subconsciously at the realization of how they are not what you thought they were and secondly, because of their modelling those same behaviours for you. Monkey see, monkey do! It's interesting to hear some teeanagers talk about themselves when they realize this... they often believe that they should somehow know how to act differently than their parents... but honestly, *how could they possibly have learned how to regulate* ***<u>their</u>*** *emotions when the people who taught them everything they know, their parents, had no clue how to regulate their own emotions?* You cannot teach someone else how to do something that you yourself have no idea how to do!

The other thing that happens when your perspective of your parents suddenly changes is that you are often left questioning everything you thought you knew about the world. If you were that wrong about your parents, then what else were you wrong about? When you no longer like your parents and therefore no longer want to be like them when you grow up, suddenly you have to figure out who you do want to be like in life. When you no longer want to be part of *their* 'herd' (i.e. group... or family), the feelings of isolation and not belonging can become intense and lead you to desperately start looking for a new herd – a group of people that will accept you and understand you – people who are ***NOT*** like your parents.[119]

So then, given that you now know what happens to most teenagers at an emotional level and why it happens, is there anything that you can do to avoid it? Do you want to avoid it? **SHOULD** you avoid it? Yes! I don't know... and yeah, it makes sense to avoid it if you can.

"... ?"

Didn't you leave yet?

"... !"

Siberia!!! Google it!

"... !!!"

OMG.... NOT CYBERIA.... S-I-B-E-R-I-A!!! Now GO!!!! HURRY!!!!!

I'm so sorry that he's part of your generation... I think that he single-handedly dropped the average IQ in this room by a good 30 points!

OK, back to the question. How can you avoid that emotional disaster (or fix it if you're already in the middle of it)? What do you need to know about your parents that will help make those feelings less intense, and eventually go away? What do you need to *understand* about them? Well, the answer to that question is actually pretty simple... simple in theory, but difficult in practice. What teenagers and young adults need to do in order to escape those feelings we just talked about is to ***build an understanding of their parents using Mini-U instead of Bob AND/OR Jim.*** However, this is

---

[119] It is this sense of no longer belonging to a parents' 'herd' and the sense of no longer believing what they believe and no longer wanting to be like them that leads most teenagers to suddenly start changing and experimenting and rebelling.

much easier said than done because Bob and Jim are going to be trying to influence them every step of the way. They will be putting thoughts into their head and answering the questions they ask themselves as they try to figure it all out.

"?"

YES!!! Exactly like the guy who just left! Except that because the statements that they make come from within their own heads, it makes it much harder to recognize that it's Jim or Bob talking. In fact, the only reliable way to tell is to double check every thought, every statement, and every conclusion that comes into your mind with your 'Dummy Detector' – Mini-U! In other words, you have to check and see if they ***make sense.*** The best way to do that is to say it (the thought or conclusion) to yourself, or to others, out loud. When you say something out loud, you force it to be processed through Mini-U. Have you ever had an idea or thought something that *you thought* made sense… right up until you said it out loud (usually when trying to explain it to someone else) and only then did you realize that it didn't really make sense?[120] Or what about when you or someone you know says something, believing that it's a fact (based on reality) but when questioned about it says that "It's really hard to explain…" and so they don't explain it… because they can't? These are all situations where Jim or Bob have 'told' us something and followed it up by assuring us that it's true and it makes sense… even though it doesn't but we accept it as true because we trust them. **DON'T TRUST THEM!!!** Force yourself to give yourself the *evidence* behind every conclusion that comes into your head. It's the only sure way of knowing that you're not making a mistake.

When teenagers are able to do this, they come to some general conclusions about their parents that help defuse those negative emotions. I could tell you what they are… but it's always best if you figure it out yourself. Nothing that anyone tells you is ever going to be as powerful as if you came to that conclusion because you figured it out yourself. So I'm going to suggest that you stop reading here. Go and think about it! Try to

[120] Ever heard someone say "That made a lot more sense in my head!"?

solve the problem on your own. Think about your parents and try and figure out what would be really important to know about them and who they are. Think of a recent fight that you had with them and see if you can understand what the fight was about, why they did what they did and said what they said. Say it out loud. Write it out. Then when you've done that come back here and keep reading and check your answers against the ones in this book.[121]

Or, if you prefer, you can just jeep on reading to find out the answers from me. If you do decide to do that, you should still go back afterwards and confirm it for yourself.

These are the answers/understandings you should have come up with.

Your parents are only human – they make mistakes... lots of them... they have made many, many mistakes and will make many, many more mistakes pretty much for as long as they live. The most important thing for your Mini-U to understand about them is that they only have a Mini-U (Logic and Reason Centre) with a volume of 4... or 3... (or even less) while their Bob (Harm Avoidance Drive) and their Jim (Pleasure Seeking Drive) are ordering them around with volumes of 10 (just like everybody else). Now, once you understand this and accept it, you will see that it means:

Most of what you have experienced with them in the past – and will continue to experience with them – is not really under their control; it happened and will keep happening because, the vast majority of the time, either their Jim or Bob is in control of their behaviours... which also means that *there probably isn't any REAL, valid "reason" for their behaviours.* This means that most of your childhood and everything that you thought you knew about life and the world and them, as people, is basically a write-off. This also means that almost everything that they have ever done or will ever do is, unfortunately, completely out of '*their*' control. To put it

[121] Just like you should do with Math homework – flipping to the back of the textbook and copying down the answers to the questions doesn't really help you understand it... but doing it and then checking the answers and, most importantly, when what you came up with is different than what's at the back of the book, figuring out *why* your answers don't match.

another way, they simply cannot stop themselves from being inappropriate and behaving the way that they do and saying the things that they say.

Given that it is pretty much a guarantee that your parents' Mini-U (Logic and Reason Centre) is very, very, very quiet, you cannot expect that they are going to "think" before they act... because they can't. So because they cannot "think" before they act, and thereby filter their behaviour, when it comes to their behaviour and its impact on you, you essentially have to do that for them. In other words, you are going to have to take **everything** that they have said and done and will continue to say and do in the future with a grain of salt (*carry a BIG bag of it...*). You will **always** have to think for yourself and figure out for yourself what parts of their interactions with you, if any, are based in reality and relevant to you!

So how do you know which pieces of information coming from them to take seriously? How can you tell what's relevant to your life, for real? How can you tell ***when*** to actually listen to them and ***when*** to actively think about what they say and do, and then filter out and ignore the crap[122]? Well, it's actually quite simple;[123] you need to start thinking about what they say and actively filtering whenever there is a lot of emotion present when they are saying/doing whatever it is that they are saying/doing – which is going to get very tiring for you because they are like that **most of the time!**

For you, the best way to do this is going to be to *ask yourself* **when YOU are not in an emotional state**, **AND/OR** *ask a friend or another adult* that you trust, if what they said/did made sense given what was going on at the time. When you are trying to figure it out, the first thing to do is to dissect the event in as much detail as you can (details help to keep it objective – based on facts) and then, when you consider ***all*** of the facts – what you ***know*** is true and real – ask yourself/friend/other adult if what your parents said or did was reasonable. If the answer to that question is "No!" then

[122] because either their Jim or Bob is in control

[123] and no different from any other teenager out there who may have been luckier than you and gotten 'average' parents – except that you will have to be thinking about the information they are presenting to you a lot more often, and then actively filtering out and ignoring a heck of a lot more crap.

the next step is to ask yourself/friend/other adult what would have been a reasonable thing to have said/done given the facts of the situation – because that's what *should* have happened.

Now, when you are asking yourself/friend/other adult these questions and trying to come up with the right answers, there are some simple 'clues' that can help guide you. The first clue to use when analyzing statements that they have made is to go over *exactly, word-for-word,* what they said. If they used the terms "always" or "never", you can stop right there 99% of the time. You see, there is a huge difference between the descriptive terms "always" and "never" (which are almost exclusively used by Jim and Bob[124]) and the terms "sometimes", "occasionally", "rarely", or "frequently" (which is Mini-U's language[125]).

The second clue to look for is the presence of any emotion at the time of the event. It's pretty easy to tell if they are feeling angry or irritated (Jim), but what about if they're feeling anxious? Or scared? Or mildly uncomfortable? Those emotions tend to be much harder to identify in parents and unfortunately, anxiety-driven (Bob-controlled) behaviour is common, but not as common as Jim-driven behaviour, for most parents. In general, if you think about the situation and the behavioural outcome was not a logical one, and you're pretty sure that they weren't "angry" at you, then it's highly likely that there was some degree of anxiety present influencing their behaviour. In general, moms are more likely than dads to have anxiety and both parents are more likely to have anxiety present when dealing with daughters than with sons.

You should also be aware that there are some parents who have **a lot** of anxiety, and it's often the only emotion present and unfortunately, it's present almost all the time. So how can you tell if one or both of your parents fit into this category? Well, generally speaking, by the time you're old enough to be reading this book, you should also be able to think about and identify (roughly) the relative volumes of your parents' Jims and Bobs. By now, you know your parents well enough to be able to identify if they

---

[124] *Remember... Jim and Bob are dumb as stumps and can't count* ☺

[125] *Because he knows how to count!* ☺

are worriers, if they get stressed easily, if they are control freaks, if they are pessimists, if they focus only on the negative, and spend most of their time pointing out what could be better, if it seems like they aren't satisfied by anything, if they seem to always have something to complain about, if they are clean freaks, etc. Parents with overly-loud Bobs (a.k.a. *worriers*) are almost always in a state of worry about something or other and will only sometimes recognize that their worrying is irrational. What this means for you is that, if one of your parents is a worrier, you should, *always* double check with your own brain (i.e. ask Mini-U) to figure out if something they are saying or doing makes any sense or not.

*******WARNING******

When you are thinking about what your parents are doing or saying, **DON'T then tell them that they are not making any sense** – that will only make the situation worse! Keep in mind that in the middle of the situation, they are not thinking rationally so to try to point that out isn't going to make any difference at all. If your Jim is pushing you, forcing you to say something, then **ONLY** ask them to explain to you how they came to that conclusion. You can say that as a way of trying to, in a roundabout way, encourage them into using their Logic and Reason Centre - if you must - but understand that *the most likely outcome of any type of challenge to what they are saying is not going to be a good one for you.* So, given that you now know this, does it really make sense to say something to them if it's not going to help change them and it's only going to hurt you???

The problem with our brain is that "Mom" and "Dad" are biologically protected from bad thoughts and negative judgements about them. Which means that even if they aren't good people and those thoughts **are** justified, if we come to those conclusions and try to keep them, we will only end up feeling angry and guilty. We will end up in a constant state of emotional turmoil because we are **not allowed to think that way about them – regardless of whether or not it is true!!!**

The best way to get around this problem is to *mentally* separate your parents into 2 parts:

" !?!?"

No, not the left and right sides...

"... ?"

OMG!!! I saw you leave!!! How did you...

"... !"

His twin brother??? You have **got** to be kidding me.... There are ***two*** of you?

"... !"

Oh, you're the *smart* one? Riiiiiiiiiiight....

"... !" "... ...." "... !" "... !!!"

....

....

"... ?"

... No... no... that was right...in fact, that was actually intelligent.... I'm sorry, I was just totally stunned to hear something smart coming out of your mouth.

"... !"

No, no.... I believe that you're the smart one now... It's just hard to believe that you two are related, let alone identical twins.

"... ..."

I'm sure that you do get that a lot. Have you ever thought of dressing a little bit differently... maybe doing your hair differently or wearing a mask or something?

"... ?"

No, no, I get it. But the fact is that he obviously isn't going to, or might just be too stupid to even know how to change. And he's walking around using your face, making your life harder because of what he's doing. So even thought "it's not fair" that you have to change what you're doing when you didn't do anything wrong in the first place, does it really make sense to continue to be judged unfairly by others because of what your brother does or says?!? If you looked different than he did, it would fix that problem.

"... ..."

Hmm.... OK. .... How about using a different icon so that we know that you aren't him from now on?

"... ... ...!!"

****

****

: "Security has arrived sir!"

Great response time guys... Did you need to bring everyone???

: "Is this the individual who needs to be removed? He fits the description you posted on Twitter!"

No, no, no, that one left already.

: "Are you certain Dr. T? He looks exactly like the picture you posted on your Facebook page... right here... the one that's tagged as *'MegaMoron'*... and the one you uploaded to your Flikr account too!"

That's because he's the twin brother of the other one.

: "A twin??? Are you sure?"

I'm sure. This one has a brain! Thanks anyways though.

: "Security... Move out! We're needed at the French-Fry riot in the Caf."

*****

So, as I was saying, sometimes, even though it's not fair, the smart thing to do to fix it yourself if you can!

"... !" → "... !"

Nice... I like it. Good choice!

OK, so then.... .... ummmm..... I totally lost my place....

"... !"

Right! Thanks. How to split your parents.

As I was saying, you want to be able to mentally split your parents' ***behaviours*** into two component parts – the good part and the bad part, and then mentally create a duplicate of your parents, each of which is going to be responsible for one of those behavioural collections. Give each of them a name and when a behaviour belonging to one of them is happening, mentally give the responsibility for that behaviour to its rightful owner.

In other words, you are going to have to think of/imagine the limited parent(s) as being two separate people – the 'good' one and the 'Screw-up' – who happen to cohabitate (both live in) a single body (just like The Hulk and Bruce Banner). Now when you picture the 'good' parent in your head, give them their face and their name but when you picture the 'Screw-up' in your head, give that version of them a different name and a different face.

"... !?!"

Exactly!!! It's almost exactly like what I suggested we do with your problem with your brother... except that both of you *really are* two separate people. For 'limited' parents, we are essentially mentally creating an 'Evil Twin' version of them to hold responsible for all of the stupidity that they send your way! We have to do this in order to fool Bob and avoid the guilt associated with thinking bad things about our 'parents'. And because we're going to be doing this to mess with Bob, *the two versions of them have to **LOOK** different!*

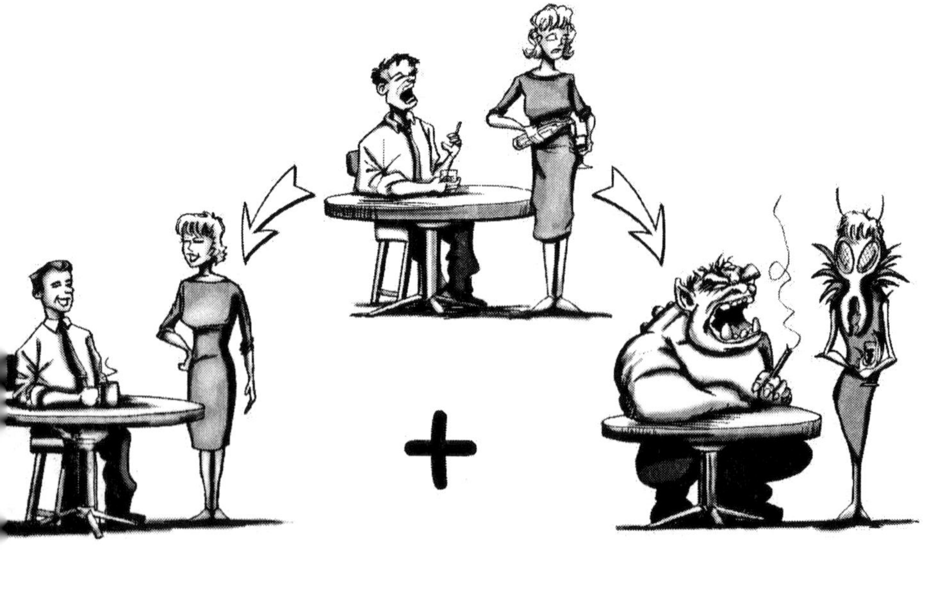

So then, once you've mentally created their Evil Twin, go and take all of your history with your parents, all of your memories of the things that they have said and done over the years as well as all of the emotional reactions you have had to them and start separating those things into 2 piles – "Good" and "Bad". Once you've done that (or, you can combine that step with the next one and sort it out as you go) give all of the stuff from the "Good" pile to the 'good' one (i.e. associate those memories and emotions to them) and give all of the stuff that's in the "Bad" pile to the "Screw-Up" a.k.a the 'Evil Twin' (associate those memories and emotions to them and *especially, all of the anger and blame* that goes along with those memories).

Basically, it's like suddenly finding out that someone does have a twin brother and it was ***him*** that was making your life miserable, not the 'good' twin. By doing this, you are essentially fooling Bob into thinking that the person that you are angry at, the person responsible for all your misery is NOT "Mom" or "Dad". Then, *because it's not them*, you are now free to be angry with (blame, dislike, hate, or otherwise think very badly about) the person responsible without any of the emotional turmoil that Bob would otherwise cause you if it *was* "Mom" or "Dad".

Now obviously, this is going to be a very lopsided distribution – with WAY MORE stuff belonging to the Screw-Up/Evil Twin and very little belonging to the 'good' parent. And that's fine – if that's what's real, then that's what's real. Luckily for you, it wasn't "Mom" or "Dad" that messed up your life and who you can't stand as a person. *nudge nudge, wink wink* And ***THAT*** is all that Bob needs to know!!!

Mini-U however needs to know one more fact – which is that even though the 'good' parent is good and everything, *they can't control when the Screw-Up/Evil Twin takes over* and so they cannot ***EVER*** be trusted about anything of importance. Your Mini-U needs to make sure that you do not put yourself at risk of being screwed over again and again by the Screw-Up/Evil Twin. You can have a relationship with your 'good' parent(s), talk to them, go visit them, whatever you want to do – just make sure that the minute the Screw-Up/Evil Twin takes over, that you aren't vulnerable – leave, stop the conversation, walk away – *do whatever you need to do to make sure that they cannot screw with your life any further.*

You are going to have to set and keep **VERY FIRM LIMITS** around your interactions with your 'good' parent(s), so that you are not continuing to put yourself at risk. It really does not make any sense to put yourself into a situation with your 'good' parent(s) where, **IF** the Screw-Up/Evil Twin took over, it could cause real problems for you[126].

You also need to recognize that you have been and will continue to be *very affected* by what happened in your childhood. Your Jim and Bob have got all sorts of crap in their databases because of your history with the Screw-Up/Evil Twin and this **WILL** have an impact on your life for the next little while – at least until you work out Mini-U to the point where he is stronger and louder than Jim and Bob.

When it comes to your parents, it is also very important for you to understand that, unfortunately, they will **always** be the way they are – *with a much louder Jim and Bob and a Mini-U that they can barely hear* – and as such, ***rarely in control of their behaviour***. Here's the good news though. The difference between you and them is that, if you decide to work out your Mini-U daily, in 2-3 years, you (Mini-U) will be in control of your behaviour rather than blindly following Jim and Bob's orders. Which means that you will not be making the same mistakes in your life as they did and continue to do... which means that you will be able to enjoy life [127] a lot more. In other words, there's still hope for you!

----

[126] For example, down the road, if you decide to see your 'good' parent(s), you should go visit them – because you can easily leave if the Screw-Up/Evil Twin shows up. Don't invite them over if it would be hard for you to kick the Screw-Up/Evil Twin out.

[127] Which is a critically important part of being happy.

Understanding your parents is not about blaming them for the mistakes and screw-ups that they have made. And it's not about figuring them out so that you can show them how to change what they are doing (because they can't). Rather, it is about recognizing that the overall low volume of their Mini-U (Logic and Reason) limits the usefulness of the information that they give you, and that most of the information/feedback that they give you (in terms of what they say and what they do) probably needs to be put aside as being useless, meaningless and false (but not in a confrontational way!).

The goal of understanding your parents is to be able to take the positive interactions and memories – no matter how few there are – that come from them and leave the negative ones behind – by minimizing/eliminating the impact of those negative ones by actively filtering them out of your head as soon as you recognize them as not being true.

Always remember that the negative interactions that come from them - that false, useless, grossly exaggerated information - is not coming from them! It's coming from their two drives (Jim & Bob) and even though they don't really mean it, they can't help it and can't stop doing it either because they aren't in control of their Jim and Bob any more than you are.

Chapter 11

Understanding Yourself

a.k.a.

When Your Drives Drive You Crazy!

The Second Hardest Task in Life – Understanding Yourself

Next on our 'To Do' list is the second hardest thing you will ever have to do... and also the one that will take the longest to complete. It is the task of understanding yourself. These next couple of chapters are all about you! Explaining yourself to you and giving you specific tips on how to manage life when your Jim and Bob are driving you crazy.

Generally speaking, there are two situations that cause problems for people when it comes to their Drives and the Drives' respective volumes:

#1 when Bob is too loud (a.k.a. when Jim is too quiet).

#2 when Jim is too loud (a.k.a when Bob is whispering).

Keep in mind that we are born with a certain baseline volume for both Jim and Bob. Most of the time, Jim and Bob's volumes are going to hover around that baseline volume but there will be times, as we go through life, depending on the situations we find ourselves in, that the respective Jim and Bob volumes will fluctuate dramatically... and catch us by surprise because we don't hear them *that loudly* most of the time. Also keep in mind that if Jim is really loud, then Bob is automatically going to be really quiet. Which means that when I discuss problems associated with an overly loud Jim or a too-quiet Bob, they are one and the same.

As I go along explaining the problems that typically occur in each situation, I'm describing someone who was **born** with a Jim/Bob volume 9 or more. If the average volumes of Jim and Bob[128] are a 5, then 'too loud' would be any situation where either Jim or Bob are yelling – from 7-ish up to 10. As I just mentioned, these problems can happen for one of two reasons – because you were born that way (in which case, most of your life is lived under those conditions and they cause you problems every single day of your life) or because there is a specific situation that you are in that Jim and/or Bob are responding to (in which case the problems they can cause for you are limited to those specific situations). These problems will only apply to you as much as the relative volume problem applies to you. In other words, the louder/quieter your Bob is, the more they will apply.

---

[128] In an average person, in an average, every-day situation

Those of you who have Bob volumes of more than 9 will be convinced that I have a little camera hidden somewhere in your house or that I've somehow managed to move into your head while those of you who have Bobs with volumes of 7 or 8 will believe that I know you pretty well but it's not like we're bffs or anything. Same goes for the description of people with too-loud Jims (a.k.a. a quiet Bob).

Chapter 11.Bob

Understanding Yourself

v1.67

When Bob Drives You Crazy!

When Bob IS a Blunderer – a.k.a. Bob's Born Too Loud:

What happens when Bob is a Blunderer? What does it feel like? How can you tell if this applies to you? Well, that's easy. If Bob IS a blunderer, then that means that Bob has blundered A LOT in your life. In other words, you have a lot of anxiety which means that you worry about almost everything, almost all of the time. The definition of worrying is "thinking about possible bad stuff that could happen". That means that you almost always have thoughts in your head about "***What if*** **insert bad thing that could happen here**". You might, or might not, recognize that your worries often make no sense at all. In fact, when Bob is a Natural Born Blunderer, he even tells you to worry about how much he makes you worry and wonders if all of that worrying is a sign of something bad... in other words, you sometimes worry about worrying ☹ ☹ ☹ . Up until you read this book, you probably tried to figure out *why* you worried so much and even though you definitely don't like all of the worrying, unfortunately, you can't seem to control it and cannot seem to stop it.

The worst time in your day is after you go to bed, but before you fall asleep, when it's dark and there is nothing to distract you from the worries that keep playing on that screen in your head. You have tried to tell your brain to shut up and stop thinking about that stuff – but that doesn't work. You:

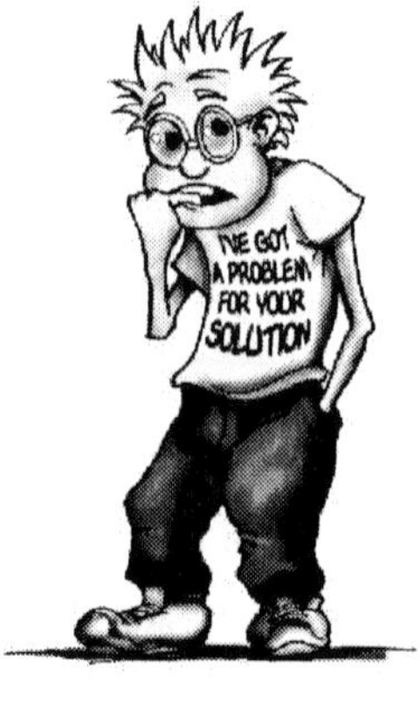

- are always predicting (or afraid that) things will go wrong.
- are mostly pessimistic and see the glass as half-empty, never half-full.
- have a very hard time relaxing and enjoying things
- In fact, sometimes, it seems like it's almost impossible for you to relax... because when you do, you start worrying... so...
- you like to try to keep yourself very busy doing something... anything.
- try to plan for everything and hate it if plans change or routines change or you have to do things differently. Most of your time and energy is

spent trying to make sure that bad stuff doesn't happen. And even when you work so hard at it and appear to have succeeded, you still have a hard time believing that everything is going according to plan... and you *feel* like things are going to go bad any second now....

- have a hard time making decisions – worried that you might make the wrong choice – even where there is no right or wrong choice.
- usually don't like new things/situations/experiences... because what if it turns out to be bad? At least, if you stick to the old stuff, what you already know, you *know* how that will turn out... you can predict the outcome[129].
- most likely have some physiologic hypersensitivities - which means that you notice (or are bothered by) tiny, little sensory experiences that most people never notice (like the tags at the back of your shirts, the feel of certain fabrics, the way clothes fit, certain sounds, certain scents, certain tastes, different food textures, etc.). You might also have many allergies – environmental allergies, drug reactions, food sensitivities (without it necessarily being a full-blown allergy). You might have a sensitive stomach and/or get a lot of stomachaches and/or headaches (for which you might have seen a doctor... or twenty... when you were younger... but they probably would have never found anything wrong that explained your stomachaches or headaches and some doctors might have even told you/your parents that it was all in your head).

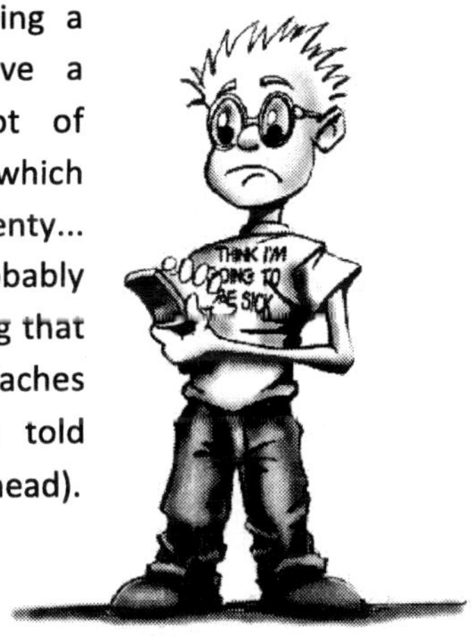

And that's not even getting into how Bob affects how you think about yourself – a.k.a. your self-esteem (it sucks) and how you think about others (you nit-pick too much, you are overly sensitive to criticism and have a hard time trusting people).

----

[129] *Have you ever noticed that you use that reasoning to justify NOT changing things and yet cannot use that same reasoning to stop worrying about the outcome even when it's the same situation over and over and over again? Kinda makes you feel crazy sometimes eh?*

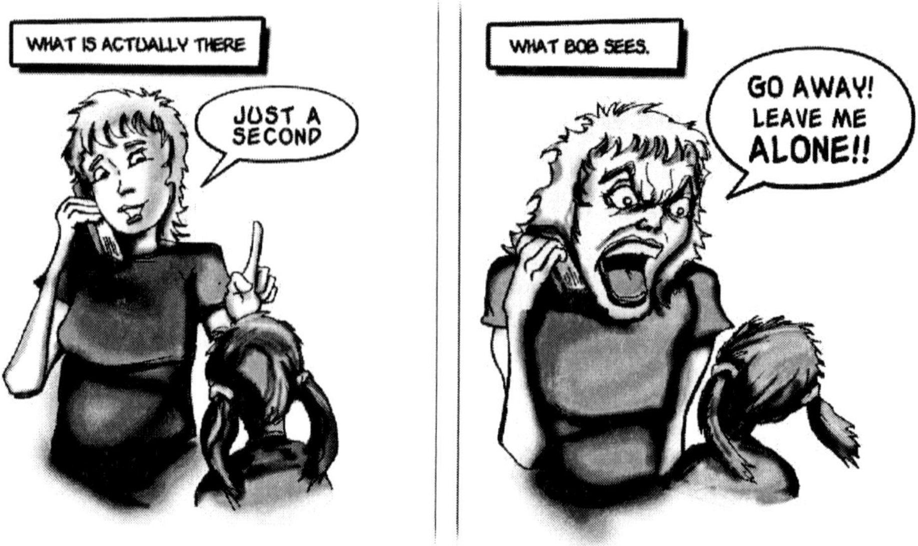

When Bob Blunders a Bit – i.e. He's Too Loud About Some Things:

As opposed to when Bob freaks out about everything… all the time (like "OMG, what if I forget to think?" or "OMG!!! There's a **tornado** warning!!!" or "OMG… GERMS!!!" or "OMG… what if mom/dad/boyfriend got into a car accident and that's why they are 2 minutes late?!?"[130]), sometimes Bob only freaks out easily about some specific stuff like 'social' stuff (i.e "what if they don't like me?" or "what if I say something stupid and embarrass myself?"[131]) or 'health' stuff (i.e. "What if I get cancer and die?" or "What if this <u>*insert physical sensation/symptom of choice here*</u> means that I'm having a heart attack or am going to die?"[132]). And sometimes, it not about any specific *group* of things, it's only about specific situations. These types of Bob-Blunders are much more common and experienced to some degree by most people. In other words, almost ***everyone*** *knows what it feels like when Bob blunders.*

---

[130] Generalized Anxiety Disorder

[131] Social Anxiety Disorder

[132] Hypochondriac

Now, there are a couple of different ways that you could end up experiencing some... or millions... of Bob-Blunders. The most common reason people end up with Bob-Blunders is because Bob's *"Danger Recognition and Recording Module"* (DRRM) is super-sensitive. The DRRM is the part of Bob that monitors your body for unpleasant body states and then, when it senses one, takes a snapshot of the environment and pastes that into the database of *Bad Stuff*. When the DRRM is super sensitive, minor, even trivial unpleasant things (like a booboo or an owwie) are sensed as being ***MAJORLY HUGE*** and therefore *all* possible causes of that booboo/owwie get recorded by that snapshot and stuck into your brain's *Bad Stuff* database.

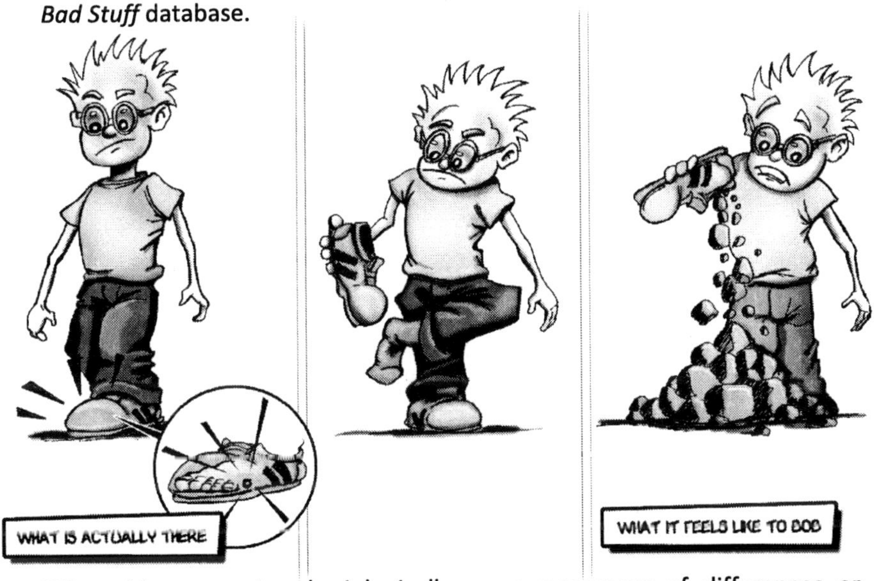

What this means is, physiologically, your awareness of differences or changes in your body states is hyper-acute. Or, to put it another way, you are aware of/can sense things (tiny, little, insignificant things) that other people do not sense to the same degree, if at all[133]. You are bothered by sensory inputs that other people don't even notice.

As a result of this hypersensitivity to your environment (both internal [your body] and external [everything around you]), when one of these

[133] You can feel (on your skin) things other people do not feel, smell things others don't smell, taste things others don't taste, see things other's don't see, or hear things others don't hear.

unpleasant body sensations/states is detected by Bob, just about anything and everything that is happening around you gets written in to your list of *Bad Stuff*... which means that your list of *Bad Stuff* is **way too big** and has lots of things on it that should not be there (because they aren't ***really, for-real-for-real*** bad or dangerous and aren't really related to whatever "bad thing"[134] your body sensed). When you have a super-sensitive Bob that identifies and records just about anything and everything into your brain's list of *Bad Stuff* and your list of *Bad Stuff* grows out of control to include just about everything, we (doctors) call this "Generalised Anxiety Disorder".

Sometimes, the stuff that ends up on your *Bad Stuff* list is not as generalised and can be restricted to a particular area of your life[135] or even more specifically to a particular thing. When the thing(s) that gets added to the list are more specific, we (doctors) call it a specific 'anxiety disorder' (if it's not one thing but rather, a cluster of related things) like Social Anxiety Disorder, or Obsessive-Compulsive Disorder, or a "phobia" like Triskaidekaphobia[136], arachnophobia[137], coulrophobia[138], or phobophobia.[139]

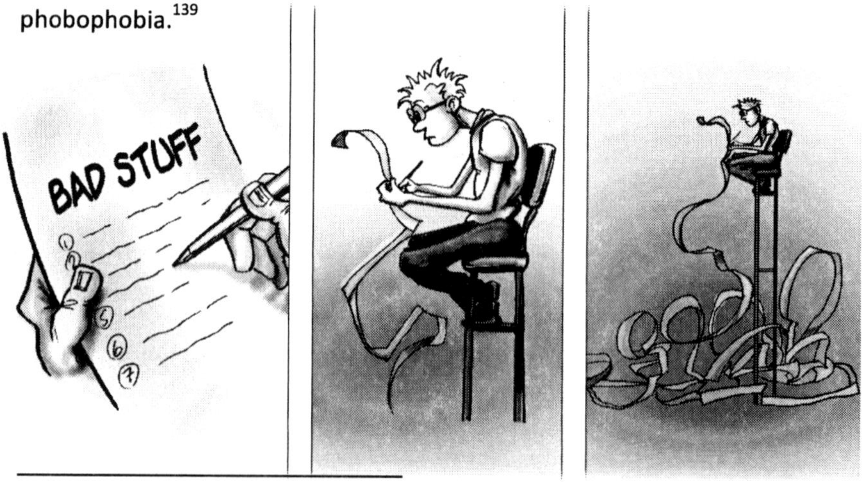

[134] If it was even a bad thing to begin with...

[135] such as your social world, the 'world' world (weather, disasters, etc.), or your own internal world (i.e. germs, illness, death, etc.).

[136] Fear of the number 13

[137] Fear of spiders

[138] Fear of Clowns

[139] Fear of Phobias

Now remember... (from wayyyyy back in Chapter 3) the reason that Bob is the way he is is because of Genetics. Bob's super-sensitivity is not something that you developed over your lifetime, or something that you mysteriously got one day, it is part and parcel of your genetic makeup (just like the colour of your skin, your eye colour, hair colour, height, etc.). It probably comes from one or both of your parents and if it's not from them, then I guarantee you that somewhere in your genetic family tree, there is some family member(s) with significant anxiety (i.e. grandparents, aunts, uncle or whatnot).

Not everyone who ends up experiencing a Bob-Blunder has a genetically super-sensitive Bob. Some people have perfectly normal Bobs and suddenly have something go wrong – either in their brains or in their lives/environment, that changes their Bob's sensitivity (sometimes, only temporarily, other times, permanently). Then, because of this 'short-circuit' in their Bob, end up having some thing(s) put into the *Bad Stuff* Database by mistake. The different ways that this can happen... don't really matter[140]... because at the end of the day, it doesn't really matter how you got here – just that you did.

The common problem for people with Bob-Blunders is that stuff that shouldn't be in the database of* Bad Stuff *is.

If this is you, it's important for you to understand that there are actually two problems here:

1) The specific thing that is mislabelled as "*Bad Stuff*" (which will apply to everyone that is in this group).
2) The problem of the supersensitive Bob (which will apply to most of you reading this though there might be a few of you with normal Bobs).

[140] *Well, that's not really true... there is one reason that this sometimes happens that is relevant to you - smoking marijuana - getting high on pot sometimes triggers and over-activates Bob... and sometimes, it does this in a very permanent way. You know that 'paranoid feeling' some people get when they are high? That's what this is... and it's very sad when an otherwise normal teenager becomes paranoid and anxious for the rest of their lives because of a bad decision. Sometimes, it happens after the first time, but sometimes it happens even after they have been smoking up for years without any 'problems'.*

This means that even if you manage to get things moved out of the *Bad Stuff* list and into the *Good Stuff* list [i.e. fix problem #1](something that I am going to explain how to do shortly), problem #2 will still be there. And unfortunately, *you can't "fix" Bob*! Yes... unfortunately, you will ALWAYS end up with stuff getting added to your list of *Bad Stuff* inappropriately[141] down the road... no matter what. This is why it's so important, especially for those of you born with a super-sensitive Bob, to have a loud, powerful Mini-U.

Without a loud/powerful Mini-U overriding what Bob is telling you to do, you will always be at the mercy of Bob's hypersensitivity and his ridiculously long and over-inclusive list of Bad Stuff.

Ideally, you will learn how to control Bob by using Mini-U. But even when this isn't the case (i.e. you do not get Mini-U loud enough or you are dealing with your own kids down the road who do not have Mini-U or you are trying to manage your parents who are living in your basement after they end up losing their mental faculties), don't worry! There is still the "fix problem #1" solution you can rely on which you can use to erase stuff from anyone's list of *Bad Stuff*; but it takes a lot of work every single time you do it. Without a loud Mini-U, you are going to have to work a heck of a lot harder as your life will be a recurrent series of these situations.[142] On the other hand, if you take the time now to train Mini-U and build up your 'willpower', then it really doesn't matter what's put on the list of *Bad Stuff* because the louder you train Mini-U to be, the more quickly and easily you

[141] by 'mistake' (these are "Bob's Blunders")

[142] Identifying something on the list of *Bad Stuff* that's there by mistake and then put in the effort and spend the time and energy needed to erase it

will be able to override the behavioural orders that Bob is giving you. This is by far and away the easier way to go through life and, I think, a much better solution than to ignore Mini-U's development now and then have to deal with Bob's Blunders for the next sixty years of your life.

Work hard now (for the next couple of years), training Mini-U to be louder than Bob so that, down the road, you won't have to work hard dealing with Bob-Blunders for the rest of your life.

I must warn you that there is another problem that can also happen to you when you have a super-sensitive Bob but it only happens once Mini-U joins the game. Once Mini-U starts observing what you are doing and noticing your behaviour and the fact that it doesn't make any sense, and the fact that you are doing things that you know are dumb, and the fact that you are freaking out about things that you know are irrational, Mini-U comments on this. This then triggers Bob, who starts freaking out about this behaviour that he is making you do! Bob then starts catastrophizing and saying all sorts of bad stuff about you because of what you are doing, and thus makes you feel guilty for doing what he told you to do in the first place.

Basically the situation is this: Bob tells you to do something (i.e. "Jump!") and you listen to Bob and you jump. Mini-U sees you jumping and says, "That was dumb! Why did you jump?". Bob hears Mini-U say this and then joins in and calls you an idiot for jumping (something he told you to do in the first place) and tells you to stop jumping. And then three seconds later, Bob tells you to jump again! This quickly becomes a negative cycle of self-blame which, if it goes on long enough, will eventually lead to feeling depressed and worthless.

The good news is that this cycle can be interrupted and stopped! ***IF you understand and accept that you are NOT IN CONTROL*** and cannot stop your body from doing what Bob is telling it to do then Mini-U can't criticise you and blame you for doing something that 1) you have no control over in the first place and that 2) you cannot stop yourself from doing and that 3) you are not choosing to do. Instead, Mini-U will rightfully criticise Bob for the stupid things he is making your body do. And if Mini-U does not criticise or find fault with *you*, then Bob is not going to have anything to react to himself.

The feeling of guilt is Bob's reaction to Mini-U's condemning stance to yourself. When you stop blaming yourself and criticising yourself and accept that, yes, you are (your body is) doing these things and no, it is not your fault, and yes, you can change it, then you will break the cycle and be in a much better position to tackle Bob head-on and build-up Mini-U so that he becomes stronger than Bob down the road. Even better though, once you understand that Bob is NOT "You", then the situation you find yourself in becomes one of "someone else trying to control you"... a situation that usually upsets Jim (makes you feel angry) which means that he is going to jump in and *help you* fight Bob. So now, automatically, you are **using a Drive to fight a Drive!!!**

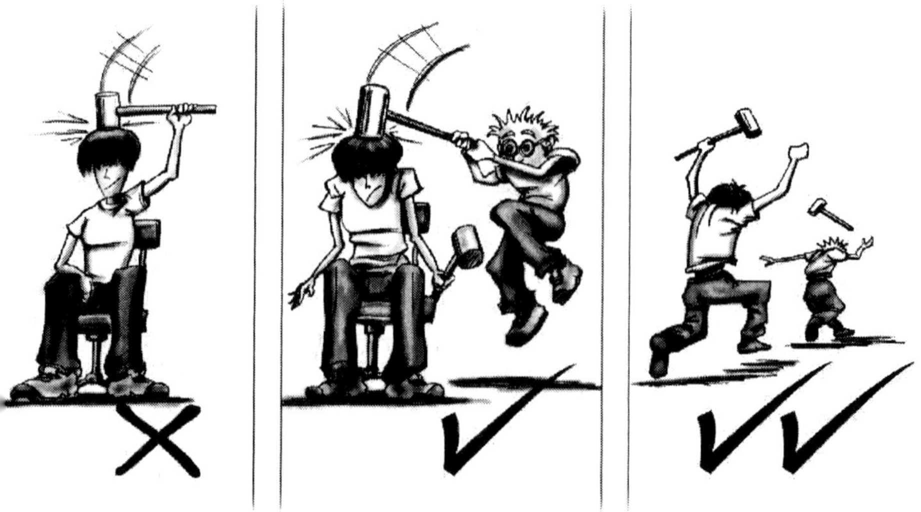

THE FIX:

So then, what do you need to do to build up the volume of Mini-U? Well, the steps are actually fairly simple, but doing it is a long-term process. The steps in building up Mini-U are the following:

1. When Bob tells you to do something, STOP and THINK about it and analyse the situation using Mini-U, and decide for yourself whether or not what Bob is telling you to do makes any sense at all. Sometimes (rarely) what Bob is telling you to do will actually make sense and is a good idea, in which case, go ahead and do it. The majority of the time, however, what Bob tells you to do will make no sense. Then go to Step 2.

2. Try really, really, really hard not to do whatever it is that Bob is telling you to do. Put it off for as long as you can. Fight him. This is what we call "using your willpower". Now, you need to understand and accept that even though you will be trying really hard, ***you will lose***. Bob *will* quickly get louder and he *will* get to be loud enough to override Mini-U and make you go and do the stuff that he wants you to do... *for now*. And that's ok because it doesn't matter if he wins - ***it's the fighting and the struggling against Bob and resisting him as long as you can that is the exercise that makes Mini-U bigger and stronger.***

   It's like weightlifting – if you want to be able to bench-press 250lbs and you start going to the gym to achieve this goal, if the very first day at the gym you put yourself down under the weight bar that has 250lbs on it and lift, you will not succeed. It is impossible to do that. You have not built up enough muscle fibres in your arms and chest (i.e. physical strength) to be able to move that amount of weight... yet. Now if you look at the fact that you could not lift 250lbs right away as a failure, and so you give up and quit going to the gym, convinced that you will never be able to lift that weight... you will be right, you never will get to that point because you didn't do the work you needed to do to get there. Everybody knows that you have to start with a weight that, with some effort, you *can* lift,[143] and then you go and you do that repeatedly, every

[143] And there will be different starting points for different people, depending largely on the natural size of their physical body.

day. If your starting point is 50lbs, and you go in every day and lift 50 lbs 30 to 50 times a day, you'll soon reach the point where lifting 50lbs takes minimal-to-no effort. That is when you increase the weight, slap on another 10lbs, and start lifting again. Most people will be able to move up about 10lbs in weight every two to four weeks because it takes that long to build up enough muscle fibres to physically be able to lift that weight.

The same thing applies to learning how to play Rachmaninov's Piano Sonata #1 or Beethoven's Sonata No. 29 on the piano – you won't be able to do it as a beginner – you have to be much more skilled and have developed your hand coordination and fine motor control through several years of regular (daily) practice in order to succeed.

It is no different for the development of the brain's neural circuitry used to control your behaviour a.k.a building up Mini-U's 'mental muscles'.

If you are an average teenager, and you are starting out at about age 16 to do this, to exercise Mini-U regularly, it will take you about 18 months to 2 years to get Mini-U to a point where he can have a relative volume of 11 or 12 and is able to override Jim or Bob whenever you want. The harder you push yourself – in other words, the more often you can remember to think and try to override whatever Bob or Jim are telling you to do, and the longer you remain in control of your behaviour, refusing to listen to them, the faster you will develop Mini-U's strength.

It takes a bit of time to get used to the idea that you are supposed to question every thought that pops into your head about what to do in any given situation. But the fact is that that is exactly what you want to do and where you want to end up at since it is much easier to intercept Jim and Bob's messages when they are just thoughts, before they get louder and become feelings. Unfortunately, even though this is the easiest point at which to intercept them, most people can't start here since it is soooo not what they have done all of their lives. What I suggest doing as a simple starting point is to simply make a ***RULE*** for yourself ahead of time that states ***'I will NOT do things that I KNOW do not make any sense to do!'*** and then try to stick to it.

In essence, whenever you have a feeling, an internal state change, a change in your mood, or you find yourself thinking that you 'feel like' blah blah blah, try to *think* – identify ***what behaviour*** is the feeling pushing you to do. That *feeling* should be the cue or trigger for you to question yourself and ask yourself "Does what the feeling is telling me to do make sense to do, yes or no?". Believe it or not, if **all** you do is to simply remember to ask yourself that question whenever you have a feeling then you will be doing enough work in order to slowly build up the strength of Mini-U. If you do more than that and try to stick to the rule you made for yourself, Mini-U will get stronger faster.

You always want to try to ask that question early on in the feeling because at that point, Bob is already pretty loud. If you find that you can't remember to ask yourself the question at that point, then, because of the *rule* you made, when you notice that you are doing stuff that makes no sense to do, *BOB* will often ask the questions for Mini-U – because Bob does not like to break rules... breaking rules is bad!!! At this point, Mini-U's job is to try to stop your 'self' from doing these behaviours (and the funny thing is that Bob will also be helping you fight his control of your 'self' as well).

If you're a real keener, and you really want to work on this hardcore, then the best way to do that is to wake up and first thing in the morning ask yourself the question, "Why am I doing this?" and then answer it. With every single thing that you do as you go throughout your day, every step of the way, force yourself to answer that question. If you cannot answer it or your answer does not makes sense, then do something else (ideally, something that makes sense to do) to change the routine of your life. Change the pattern, in any way, because that will be YOU overriding what Bob or Jim are telling you to do.

Keep in mind that this is a very tiring thing to do. Using Mini-U is exhausting work. Our brains actually use up the better part of 1/3 of all the energy requirements of our body and studies have repeatedly shown that the simple act of *'exercising willpower'* significantly drops blood sugar levels.[144] Once again, it is exactly like working out. If you want to go hardcore and work out for an hour a day, seven days a week, you will start to see the benefits of working out and the changes in your body much faster than someone who simply works out for half an hour, three to four times a week. But you will also be much more tired and physically exhausted because of all that extra work that you are doing.

Most people cannot maintain this level of mental exercise for an extended period of time, and so I recommend that you simply try to do it in moderate amounts in an on-going manner. If some days you want to push yourself and go all-out, that's fine, but don't expect to be able to do this every day, all day, for months. It simply won't happen. If you expect that you can and then try and fail, then Bob will probably start to criticise you for not having succeeded and for having quit, and failed, and on and on and in the long run (or the short run), that isn't going to help Mini-U get to where you want to be.

---

[144] The sugar in your blood is your body's energy source, and as you do stuff that requires energy (i.e. work, exercise, thinking) it gets used up – just like gas in a car. To refill it, you have to eat.

Chapter 11.Jim

Understanding Yourself

V 2.35

When Jim Drives Drive You Crazy

a.k.a

"Life Without Bob"

a.k.a

"How to Die Young"

Jim: "What the... HOW DARE YOU talk about me second... I should be FIRST!!!"

When Jim is TOOOOOOOOOO loud and won't shut up!!!

Once again, problems with Jim come in two varieties: the kind that you are born with (a.k.a 'life without a Bob') and the kind that come up as a result of situations in our lives where, even though we aren't born that way, right then and there, when it comes to that specific thing, Jim is in full control of our behaviour. I'm going to discuss people whose lives are entirely controlled by Jim first and then move onto discussing those born with a normal Bob.

Are you 'Born without a Bob'[145]? How do you know if this is you? Other terms that are often used to describe this population include "Alpha Male", "Boss Dog", "Leader of the Pack". So then, is this you? Well, the fact is that it's highly unlikely to be you... because people whose lives are completely controlled by Jim have certain characteristics that, in general, apply to almost all of them. Some of the main characteristics that cause problems are that they do not ever believe that there is anything wrong with them or what they do, and they believe that they already have all the answers to everything. In other words, I would be very pleasantly amazed if they were reading this book and got to this point in it.

Now, just to make sure that we're talking about the right kinds of teenagers, let me describe a '*typical*' **Alpha**. In one sentence, it would be this: "You are always getting into trouble!" You...

- always have to have it your way and don't stop until you get what you want
- can't stand people trying to tell you what to do – especially if they tell you that you **have to** do it
- could care less about what others want if it doesn't match what you want
- don't really care about what other people think about you... as long as they think about you.

[145] It's not really 'without' a Bob... more like your Bob is in the bottom 5th percentile in terms of possible volume – the vast majority of the time, you don't hear him at all.

Jim: "What the... HOW DARE YOU talk about me second... I should be FIRST!!!"

- love being the center of attention and go out of your way to get it
- believe that rules were meant to be broken or at least bent or bypassed
- are intensely competitive and always want to win at everything
- aren't really bothered by much in life... except being bored... which you **hate**... which kinda sucks because you
- get bored with things (activities, people, relationships) very quickly
- have a very fast, very intense temper that can turn on a dime
- are impatient and want everything to happen right now. You can't stand waiting
- always want something else, something new or something different. You rarely feel satisfied ('happy') with your life and always want **MORE**
- are willing to try anything (just for the hell of it)
- are very stubborn/determined/insistent
- feel justified in just about anything that you do (or can find a way to justify just about anything...)
- rarely feel guilty for things that other people feel guilty over
- would love to have that T-shirt that says "as a matter of fact, it **IS** all about me!" since that's your motto in life[146]
- etc., etc., etc.

Now, on the off chance that one of you is reading this chapter, and is willing to *think*... I'll fill you in on what you need to know if you want to succeed in life... because the other simple fact is that for teenagers like you, there are only two outcomes for your life:

1. You will end up ridiculously successful in life. You will be rich and/or famous and/or powerful and/or influential – a president or CEO of a corporation, an elite athlete, a millionaire or some other variation of a very prestigious, successful life...

OR

2. You will end up in jail and/or dead before your time.

[146] This is what people call self-centered.

<u>Jim: "What the... HOW DARE YOU talk about me second... I should be FIRST!!!"</u>

There are no other outcomes for you. You will never be satisfied with an average, everyday sort of life – going to work for someone else, having to do what others tell you to do all the time and following all of the rules that would get you a comfortable, 'normal' life. And if you are still reading this, then you have the potential to be in category #1 because you are willing to think.

Another way to understand/think about it is by using the following analogy:

> *If life is a road and our bodies are cars on that road, your car came off the assembly line with the gas pedal floored and brakes that don't work. Your Jim is incredibly powerful because it has nothing to slow it down or hold it back. Your car stops for nothing and no one. You are both lucky and unlucky at the same time. Because you have no brakes, you will be able to go places and do things and achieve in life what few other people can... or... because you have no brakes, you will crash against the side of a mountain or go flying off the edge of a cliff or... I'm sure that you get the picture.*

Yes, you will get to wherever you are going in life much faster and much more easily than others out there... but ***<u>ONLY IF YOU LEARN HOW TO STEER!!!</u>*** *Thinking* – using Mini-U – is the equivalent of steering.

IF YOU DO NOT PUT YOUR HANDS ON THE STEERING WHEEL, IT IS NOT A QUESTION OF IF YOU WILL CRASH AND BURN... IT IS ONLY A QUESTION OF <u>WHEN</u>!!!

What this means for you is that you had better learn how to steer if you want to win in life. *<u>**This is where Mini-U comes into play!**</u>* You need to know that your life ***will NOT*** go OK if you refuse to put your hands on the steering wheel. Sure, it might be fun... but it will be very short. The Alphas who succeed in life are the ones that learned how to steer. Those that didn't learn... well... they didn't succeed.

Jim: "What the... HOW DARE YOU talk about me second... I should be FIRST!!!"

THE FIX:

This is the same as the fix for people with loud Bobs except that for you, it's going to be Jim that you are fighting, not Bob. Unfortunately for you, Jim is tougher than Bob!

Because Jim is so tough to beat, you need to become an expert in knowing how to *use a Drive to fight a Drive* – specifically, how to use Jim against Jim. For Alphas, the single most important thing that they can have in their life is ***A GOAL*** – something that they really, really, really want to have or to acheive – something that they have decided is worth it to work towards. Then they need to remind themselves of that goal in a visual/auditory/sensory way every day, as soon as they wake up in the morning, before Jim really gets going. And when Jim is about to make them do something stupid... something that will/might get in the way of them getting what they want, they need to remember to ask themselves this specific question – "What do I want more... this (the stupid thing) or (the long-term goal that is really important to them)?" – word for word, out loud if they can – and then give themselves the answer (again, out loud is best!). The reason for doing this is to hopefully, distract Jim from the current stupid thing that he wants and redirect him back to that appropriate, long-term thing that he also wants... *more*.

Olympic athletes can only achieve their incredible level of mastery because they are willing to do whatever it takes to get that Gold Medal. They train every day and surround themselves with pictures of the Gold Medals, the podiums, the goals so that they can stay focussed on it day in and day out. Always have a goal... and if you don't have one, then find one or make one. You need a destination so that you can steer in the right direction. After all, if you don't know where you are going, then what does it matter if you steer or not? If that doesn't work, and you are still following Jim instead of Mini-U, then the next best thing is to continue to try to activate Jim against Jim, but to use something that is much more immediate (and thus, more relevant to Jim). In order to do this, ask yourself (out loud is always best) if you are really that pathetic and that weak-willed and so completely helpless, incapable and unable to control yourself... are you really just a two year-old in an adult's body??? Really...?[147]

The reason you should be using these words is that you want to get Jim's attention and make him change his focus from whatever he is currently fixated on to *proving those statements wrong*. An Alpha's Jim *knows* full well that none of those statements are true! It *knows* that it is powerful, competent, and has all the characteristics of a natural leader! If anyone ***ever*** dared to say that kind of stuff to him, dared to imply that he was anything less than Number One... well then, he would just have to go and kick the crap out of them and show them who's boss! So then, if he has to make you ***not*** smoke a cigarette, or ***not*** get into a fight with someone, or ***not*** steal that thing, or ***not*** break the rules... then he will... just to prove a point!!!

Besides which, it is actually true! Think about it for a second... if all the guy who is talking trash about you or calling you out or egging you on has to do is say something and as a result, you ***HAVE TO*** fight back... because you ***CAN'T JUST WALK AWAY***... then, in fact, **HE IS CONTROLLING YOU!!!** If you *cannot decide to* walk away, to say nothing, then **you are weaker than him!!!** Winning is not about who can physically hurt someone else... it's about who can *control* someone else. Who cares if you pound him because of what he said? If the guy at school *wanted* you to do that in the first place so that he could have you charged and have a restraining order placed on you and therefore *force you out* of your school... then he wins! The guy with the real power is not the guy that fights... it's the guy that makes others fight! If you knew that, in order to win, you had to let someone punch you in the head... and that after they hit you, ***because they hit you***, then they would be totally screwed and they would lose... be humiliated, embarrassed and completely lose all of their street cred ... you would do it. You know you would!

----

[147] If you are NOT an Alpha, DO NOT DO THIS!!!

Jim: "What the... HOW DARE YOU talk about me second... I should be FIRST!!!"

Temporary Jim Take-Overs

This section is for everyone else who has to deal with temporary Jim take-overs in their lives. Jim take-overs are those times when Jim's craving for Dopamine is so intense that he takes over control of our bodies and blocks out Bob so that all we can hear is him telling us what to do to get him what he wants... to get him his Dopamine. Jim take-overs are very common and happen to everyone. In fact, the louder your Jim is relative to your Bob, the more often Jim is going to take-over. How can you recognize a Jim take-over? Easy! If you are *actively doing something* that does not make sense to do – *going out of your way to get something* it is probably a Jim Take-Over.

When Jim takes over, we do things that we should not do... over and over and over... even though we *know* that we shouldn't be doing them. Most of the time, Jim Take-overs involve us *doing* stuff that we shouldn't be doing – in other words, they are *active* mistakes we are making and they make up the vast majority of the mistakes that people make in their lives. ...Which makes learning to control Jim – in order to stop him from taking over – very important!!!

Now, even after you manage to train your Mini-U to the point where you are stronger/louder than Bob and Jim, there will still be times in our lives when we are at the mercy of Jim and Bob. Because Mini-U needs energy to function, when those energy reserves[148] go down for whatever reason, Mini-U's strength is drained – he will be weaker and could even end up completely incapacitated. During those times, we, once again, end up being in the position of *only* having Jim and Bob in control of our behaviour.

---

[148] Energy reserves are slowly used up throughout the day – every minute that we are awake uses some up. 'Tired' means that our body is running out of energy. Energy only goes into the system when we eat (a little, immediate boost) and when we sleep (refills the longer-lasting energy tanks). The more 'tired' or 'hungry' you are, the harder it is for you to *think*. We are at our worst emotionally and make more behavioural mistakes late at night when we are tired and/or hungry than we do in the mornings and early afternoons.

Jim: "What the... HOW DARE YOU talk about me second... I should be FIRST!!!"

The most common situations in life in which Jim is most likely to take-over include (but are not limited to):

- **GETTING MAD – LOSING YOUR TEMPER**
- Smoking cigarettes/weed
- Using recreational drugs
- Gambling
- Playing games with others
- Eating
- Playing computer/video games
- Surfing the net (especially online chatting / Facebooking)
- Dating (physical/emotional attraction to someone)
- Shopping
- Sex
- Driving

What these things have in common is that they are under Jim's control to begin with. They are things that we ***like*** – things that release Dopamine in our brains. And since Jim starts out in control, he often stays in control while we are engaged in that activity. And if Jim *really likes it...* if it releases a lot of Dopamine, he will want to keep going and going and going and going – just like the energized-by silver batteries bunny. It is when we are in these situations that we often end up making mistakes... doing things or behaving in ways that could hurt us and/or could bring bad things into our lives – making mistakes of over-indulgence or making mistakes of just plain stupidity.

A mistake of over-indulgence is when we are doing something that is not inherently bad or wrong... except that we end up doing it way TOO much or for way TOO long. This includes things like:

- Over-eating/bingeing and/or snacking on those high calorie sweets... like ***CHOCOLATE....mmmmmmm.....*** [149]
- Watching TV, surfing the net, chatting on the phone, messaging/texting or playing video games for too long (i.e. staying up

[149] *Oh great... now I just activated a craving for that huge, two pound bar of Dark Chocolate that's sitting on the top of my fridge... it's very, very..... VERY good chocolate... ... ... so it's a darn good thing I have it hidden from myself!!!*

really late to do it and therefore not getting enough sleep) or when you should be doing something else (instead of studying for a test or doing homework or listening to the teacher or interacting with people in RL[150])

- Drinking at all (unless you are of legal age) or too much (getting so tanked that you don't even remember the great time you supposedly had)
- Liking someone... and because of that, breaking rules, lying to people, getting into bad situations, or ***allowing yourself to be treated badly by the person you like...*** in order to be around them and to get their attention.
- Sex – with the wrong person or at the wrong time or in the wrong place or unprotected.
- Getting pressured into doing stuff that you wouldn't normally do so that people/friends/peers like you.
- Spending way more than you can actually afford to spend.
- Speeding down the highway at anything over 20km/h over the limit.
- Getting into fights because you don't want to let anyone get away with talking smack about you
- Being stubborn to the point of costing you... to prove a point
- Etc.

A mistake of just plain stupidity is when Jim makes us do something that we shouldn't be doing ***at all*** and is just a stupid thing to do... at all... ever... even just a little bit. This includes (but is not limited to) things like:

- Stealing/shoplifting/"borrowing it"... indefinitely... without the owner being aware that you borrowed it
- Hitting someone, for any reason, under any circumstances (unless in self-defence)
- Being mean[151] to people and/or animals
- Smoking

---

[150] Real Life

[151] Being 'mean' means purposely hurting others with words or actions

Jim: "What the... HOW DARE YOU talk about me second... I should be FIRST!!!"

...and in a section all on its own since it is so relevant to your lives...

USING RECREATIONAL DRUGS

There is one thing that is ***really, REALLY important*** for you to understand about Jim take-overs: they come in two varieties: the kind that you **WILL NOT** be able to handle[152] and the kind that you **WILL** be able to handle. What goes into which category depends on how much Jim likes that thing – in other words, how much Dopamine gets dumped into your brain when you are exposed to it the ***First Time***. The more dopamine that is dumped, the harder it will be to control.

ANY 'addictive' substance is addictive because it forces the release of **lots** of dopamine in the brain. In order to help explain the effect that drugs have on the brain, I'm going to use two analogies – money and sound – both represent Dopamine levels in the brain.

In your life, there will be some things you encounter that make your brain buzz with dopamine. This is like getting paid $50,000/day or listening to music at 120 decibels (louder than a jet taking off). The amount of dopamine released by that experience is so far above and beyond anything that your brain has ever experienced or ever will experience that it is in a class all by itself. This is not a good thing because Jim's take on this is that if that experience is available, then *nothing else in the world matters as much as that experience!* Which means that there is nothing that you will be able to find that will be able to distract Jim. If you run into one of these things in your life – things that you have absolutely no control over, then the ***ONLY*** strategy you can use against Jim is to never let him see it.[153] Recreational drugs are like that for a lot of people – they become completely addicted or hooked after the very first time they tried it. When it comes to drugs, sometimes, you don't get a second chance.

---

[152] distract Jim from his goal

[153] Don't be around it, don't look at it, don't talk about it, don't listen to people talk about it, etc.

Jim: "What the... HOW DARE YOU talk about me second... I should be FIRST!!!"

And it's not only that there is nothing that you can use to distract Jim, but the more he keeps going to that source of dopamine, the less important every other 'normal' source of dopamine becomes. If you listen to your music at 120 decibels all the time, your brain gets used to that volume such that when it stops, you can't hear anything that's played at a 'normal' volume any more. Ever notice how people who are stoned just kinda sit there, grinning, but not doing anything? Ever notice how they will sacrifice girlfriends or boyfriends if they have to choose between them and drugs? In other words, even the large amounts of dopamine that released during orgasm (the biggest 'natural' rush of dopamine there is) is not as important as getting high.

So, what about weed? I'm sure that you've heard people say that it's not addictive, right? **WRONG!!!** Marijuana does not have an associated 'physical withdrawal' syndrome (while many other addictive substances do) because the active ingredient in marijuana – the THC – gets absorbed into the fat cells of your body while you are smoking up. Then, when you are not smoking up, the THC is slowly released back into your bloodstream over a period of days to weeks (depending on how much and how often you are smoking up). A physical withdrawal syndrome happens because the body *suddenly* does not have the addictive chemical in their body any longer. With marijuana, it never *suddenly* disappears from your bloodstream. It slowly fades.

BUT – that does not mean that it is not psychologically addictive – that Jim doesn't care about it... because he does... he likes it a lot. It gives him *lots* of dopamine. But you don't notice this until it has completely left your bloodstream – which isn't for several days and sometimes, up to 3 weeks later. For someone who smokes marijuana to say that they are not addicted and prove it by not smoking up for a couple of days or a week or two is like someone who smokes cigarettes saying that they are not addicted and proving it by not smoking for 2-3 hours. That proves nothing!!! If you want to prove that you are not addicted to it, then you have to not use it for 2-3 months... minimum. And if you are not addicted to it, then why do it in the first place? It's not good for you, it costs money, it doesn't help your brain develop in any way (in fact, it does the opposite) and there are very real nasty possible side effects associated with using it – like becoming psychotic... permanently. And if you do it a lot, then the rest of life just isn't as much fun or as interesting and everything other than smoking up becomes "boring"! Why would you *want* to do that to yourself? It makes *no sense at all!!!*

Obviously, it's a given that learning to control Jim by training up Mini-U is still the best thing to do. BUT since it takes a while to get Mini-U to that point, and because of those times when Mini-U is incapacitated due to lack of energy, knowing how to ***use a Drive to fight a Drive*** is **ALSO** a very important skill to have. When dealing with Jim, we have to use Jim to fight Jim. Bob is not much of a help against Jim. Knowing how Jim works allows us to easily outsmart him and turn him against himself... after all, remember that he is as dumb as a stump!

The two characteristics of Jim that are going to be the most useful in doing this are:

1. He can only focus on one thing at a time
2. Everything in his list is interchangeable – it's all just about the Dopamine.

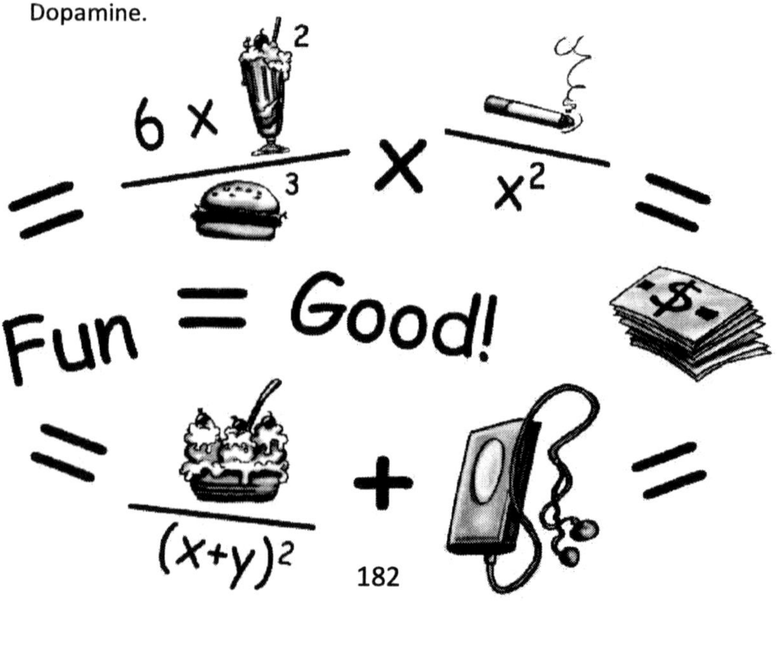

Jim: "What the… HOW DARE YOU talk about me second… I should be FIRST!!!"

Now, because of these two things, all we really need to do to effectively control Jim (if Mini-U is unable to) is to distract him with something else that he likes – find a way to get his attention unfocussed from the stupid thing by dangling something else that he also really likes right in front of his nose. This is what people automatically try to do when they are trying to quit smoking – they eat a lot of candy and chocolate. It's not about any oral fixation thing… it's about dopamine replacement. The fact is that if, instead of eating chocolate, they went to watch a movie that they have been dying to see or played a video game that they loved, or did something else that they really enjoyed, then they would be equally distracted from the nicotine craving for as long as they kept the dopamine flowing in their brain.

At the end of the day, no matter the problem, whether it's Jim or Bob, the solution is the same – it's all about building up Mini-U by working him out and using a Drive to fight a Drive if/when one of your Drives is about to beat Mini-U.

CONTROLLING YOUR TEMPER

I want to quickly talk about a very specific Jim problem – Temper! Getting angry isn't a Jim take-over per se – but all of the stuff that you *do while you are angry*[154] is. People who have problems controlling themselves while they are angry often try to justify their actions – by justifying the anger and pointing out that it was because of what the other person did that things happened – the *other person* made them mad! It wasn't their fault that they got mad… so the way to stop them from being out of control when they are mad is to make sure that other people don't piss them off!

I agree completely with the first statement – getting mad is a mental reflex of Jim's (primarily). Anger is a hard-wired, biological response from Jim

---

[154] yelling, screaming, swearing, insulting, being mean, being cruel, hitting, throwing stuff, breaking things, hurting others, etc.

<u>*Jim: "What the... HOW DARE YOU talk about me second... I should be FIRST!!!"*</u>

(like 95% of the time) or Bob (only like 5% of all anger seen in life comes from Bob). It is our ***Super Power Booster***. When Jim is responsible for the anger, it is because Jim has his sights set on something and someone or something comes in between him and what he wants... ... So, he has to become stronger, more powerful, in order to smash through whatever is blocking him from getting his dopamine.[155]

But the second part of that statement is ridiculous! It is <u>***NEVER***</u> someone else's responsibility to control *your* anger! You are the only one responsible for that... if you want to be thought of as more than just a wild animal... an actual evolved human being as opposed to a chest-thumping, club-carrying Cro-Magnon. This is one of the most important aspects of our 'self' that we need to learn to control. Fortunately, it is very easy to do... once you know how your brain works... which now you do.

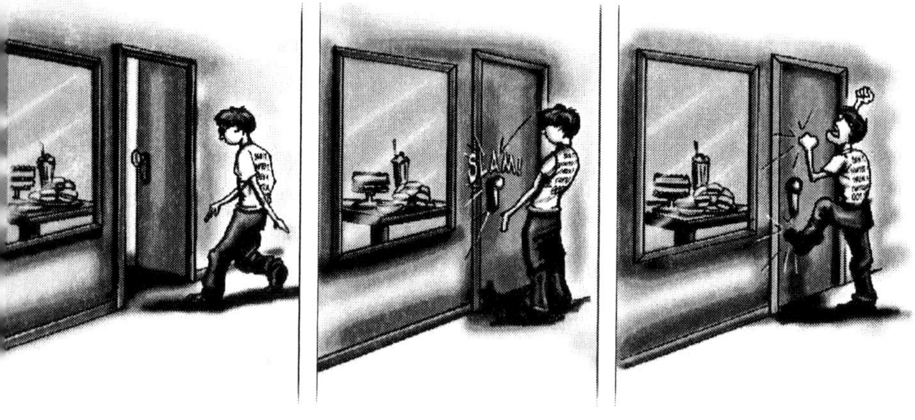

Controlling anger is best done by not getting angry in the first place – by either going <u>***around***</u> the roadblock <u>*as soon as you realize that one is there*</u> (use the thinking part of your brain to find another way to get what you want) or by using the other strategies I just explained – giving Jim dopamine from somewhere else to fool him into thinking that he got what he wanted or getting Jim to notice and set his sights on – a.k.a ***want*** – something else that he likes.... even more. When I teach parents how to

[155] because in Jim's eyes, his life depends on his 'self' getting its dopamine!

stop their children's temper tantrums, I tell them to take the thing that they know their child really, *really,* ... **reallyreallyreallyreallyreallyreally** wants and make it so that the ***ONLY*** way for them to get it is to 'NOT lose their temper' ... to remain calm. The vast majority of the time, when the parents follow through and do what I suggested, they are amazed at the fact that their child never even looked like they had to *try* to control their temper... that they weren't even getting mad any more. The reason for that is because it is exactly what it looks like → *they don't get mad in the first place...* because there is nothing stopping them from getting what they want... except their 'selves'... which they (Jim and Bob) control.

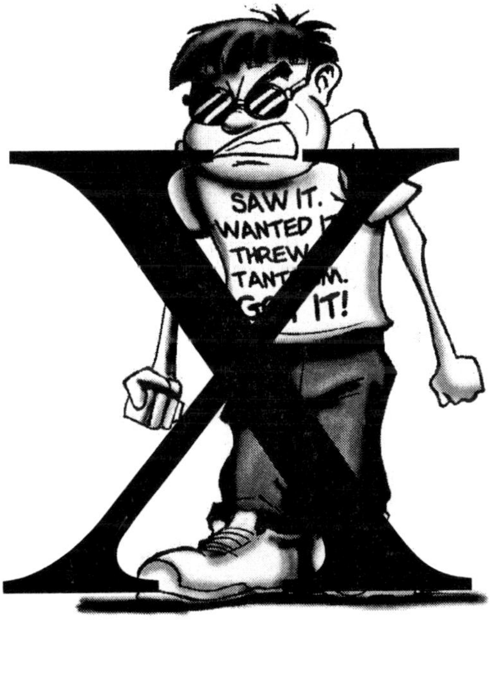

Chapter 140 km/h

"Rules of the Road"... Once You Have Hair

a.k.a.

*Things you **NEED** to know about Life*

Rules of the Road

There are three ***FACTS* or *RULES*** about *Life* that you ***need*** to know about – rules that will change everything you thought you knew about yourself.[156]

Fact #1:

You don't *really* know… you just *think* you know!

Almost everything that you think you know about life and people and the world isn't really what you know, it's what your parents (or other trusted adults in your life)…

"… ?"

or… I suppose… … … hyper-intelligent monkeys… *When did you get back???* … **sigh…** … know and have told you about life and people and the world.

Remember what we discussed back in the chapter on how we got to be here today and the critically important influence of our parents on what we know by the time we do get here? The thing is, even if you THINK that you know something for yourself, the reality is that no matter what your own post-Mini-U experiences have taught you, you interpreted those experiences through a biased filter. Your brain (i.e. Bob) wants and needs your parents to be right so he will selectively see stuff that fits what they have told you and selectively ignore information that would contradict what they've taught you.

Now keep in mind that Jim's contribution here is that he always believes that he's right about everything – including what he thinks he knows… even if it is something that he knows *only* because someone else told him so. But because of that, most of the time, we only try to prove that *WE* are right and try to prove that *OTHERS* are wrong. We rarely ever challenge our own knowledge and go about searching for evidence that proves that we are wrong!

---

156 *(There are other rules… many more than just 3… but these are the three most important ones that most people don't know and therefore cannot teach to their kids). (btw - these are the "Rules of the Road" in case you hadn't figured that out yet☺)*

Because Jim's assumption going into anything is that he is right and what he thinks is a fact, and Bob's assumption going in is that our parents are right, and what Jim knows is what our parents taught us, we end up behind the 8-ball in terms of being able to accurately see the world around us. Jim leads us to make mistakes in judgement by only seeing what supports his beliefs while Bob makes us selectively ignore stuff that would contradict our parents. As a result, we rarely ever change our minds about things that we believe about the world. Often, the only way that we change our minds is if there is SOOOOOOO much evidence against what we believe... and even then, we will often blindly feel like we are still right... somehow....

So, now that you know this, think about what it means. Does it make any sense at all to hold onto a belief and defend it so adamantly when that belief is only what someone else told us about something they believed... and the evidence contradicts it? If your father told you that the mosquitoes in Manitoba were very big and hunted in packs and would sometimes attack little dogs (like Chihuahuas) and then carry them away back to their nests to feed... and that that was why there weren't a lot of little purse dogs in Manitoba, should you insist to your teachers that it is true even when they explain to you *why* it's not possible and even show you pictures of mosquitoes from Manitoba? Logic and reason would dictate that you change your belief about Manitoba Mosquitoes... and seriously start questioning other stuff your dad has told you about... like oysters growing on trees...[157]

[157] *Not that I've ever done anything like that to my teenage daughter....*

Fact #2:

The answer to the question "Who knows you best?" isn't "Me!" (meaning you...)... it's "Everybody else!"

a.k.a.

"Objects in mirror are different than they appear to be!"

I know what you're thinking – *'Chocolate Chip cookies are really, really good.'* I agree completely – especially when you crush them and then sprinkle them on Chocolate-Butterscotch ice-cream. I know what else you're thinking – *'What the heck is this guy talking about?!?'*. You probably don't believe me... but it's true... try it! It's delicious!

"?"

Oh, sorry, I lost my train of thought there. Ummmm... right!.. like.... "Who knows you best?" Right? You want to know how I can make such an outrageous statement and then jump straight to ice-cream cookie recipes without giving you an explanation... right? OK. Here's the explanation.

People know that in order to know someone, you have to know stuff about them. And the more you know about someone, the better you know them... by definition. So when it comes to you, who else in the world could possibly know more about you than you? After all, you are with your 'self' 24/7/365. You see yourself naked and dressed and everything in between. You know the thoughts that go on in your head that you don't share with anyone! You see yourself at your best and at your worst... so how can ANYONE know you better than you know yourself?

Well, **if** that was where the facts ended and there was nothing else to say, you would be right... **but** you are missing one crucial piece of information... which is...

Oh, ummmm...... hang on....

Dang it all, I can't remember what it was …. but trust me – if you knew it, you would see how everything else doesn't matter! Trust me! … …

"… !"

OK fine… don't trust me… I'll think of it in a second… … … … … … … … … ……
… … … … … … … …… … … … … … … … …… … … … … … … … …… … … … … … …
…… … … … … … … … …… … … … … … … … …… … … … … … … … …… … … … … …
… … …… … … … … … … … … …… … … … … … … … … …… … … … … … … … …… … … …
… … … … …… … … … … … … … …… … … … … … … … … …… … … … … … … … …… …
… … … … … … … ummmmmm… … … … … … … … … …… … … … … … … … …… …
… … … … … … … …… … … … … … … … … …… … … … … … … … …… … … … … … …
…… … … … … … … … … …… … … … … … … … … …Oh wait… now I remember… it's ¾ of a cup of chocolate chips… not 3 cups…

"…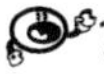?!?"

Oh wait, you're right… wrong thing I remembered! … …. …. …. What was the question again?

" !"

RIGHT!!! OK. Now I remember!

The reason why all of that stuff doesn't matter is that our brain was never designed to process information about our 'self'. *'Self'* information is automatically distorted by Jim and Bob the minute our brains try to process it, which results in a distorted perception of the experience of *'US'* (this is much the same distortion that they apply to information about the world that contradicts currently held beliefs). The result is that it's like looking into a warped mirror – the reflection that you see is not what the object really looks like… it's a twisted, distorted version of the real thing. That's what our brains do to all *'Self'* information when it comes into the brain.

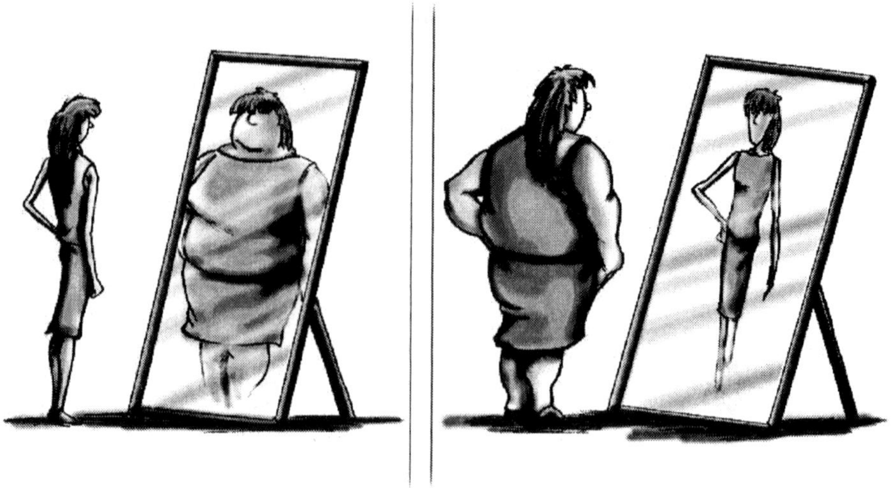

Now of course, I don't expect you to believe me right off the bat[158] – I'll prove it to you!

- Have you ever listened to a recording of yourself? Does it sound like you? I know that you don't think so but ask the people around you if it does – they will tell you it does. *The only person in the world who does not think that your voice actually sounds like your voice is YOU!!!*. No, this is not because of crappy recording devices – your voice would not sound like your voice to you even on an awesome high quality digital recorder! Try it. Record a conversation with a friend then listen to it played back – they will sound like them but you won't sound like 'you'... or at least, that's what your brain is telling you. Your brain is saying that the sound waves that are coming from that device do not match the sound waves that you have repeatedly stored (memorized) in your brain that belong to you... which is impossible since you *know* that you just said that stuff. Funny thing is, your friend will be thinking the same thing – that you sound like you but they don't sound like them. Why? Because when you hear you talking, it is '*Self*' information and as such, it is distorted and what you 'hear' is a distortion of what's really there. But when you are listening to an audio file, that's not 'self'

158 *In fact, I would be a bit disappointed if you did given how much I've been stressing the need to think for yourself and to question your world and not to simply blindly trust what you've been taught about life by others*

information... that's just sound coming from a recording device. The fact that you know that it's 'you' is why you try to match it up to what you *think you know* you sound like... but it doesn't match!

- Are you an artist? Do you know anyone who is an amazing artist and can draw people and faces very well? Have you/they ever tried to draw their own face? They can't! A Self-portrait is one of the hardest things in the world to draw – because what we see when we are drawing doesn't match the image that we have in our heads of what we look like. It's sort of close-ish... but it simply doesn't match. In fact, it can never match the image in our heads.

- Have you ever seen a picture of yourself that you thought looked **exactly** like you? Not one that you were happy with (because you thought it made you look better than you really are) but one that you thought looked **exactly like you**! Again – go through a bunch of pictures with friends and ask them to pick out some of the pictures that they think look exactly like you – then look at the ones they chose – you probably won't agree with them. Again, *you are the only one out there that sees your face the way you do... distorted!* Everyone else out there sees it far more accurately than you do.

- Look around you at everyone you know – how many of your friends who think they are fat but are really not fat, who think they are ugly but are really attractive, who think they are geniuses but really they're idiots, who have amazing singing voices but think that they suck, who believe they are god's gift to men/women but really... they aren't, who think they look awesome in those muffin-topping jeans but really... well, seriously??? And of course, when you see them walk by, you think to yourself *'Did they NOT look in a mirror this morning??? Like... OMG!!!'*
  The problem is that they did – and unfortunately, what they saw reflected back in their brains was a distorted version of reality. Sometimes this distorted image is better than what's real and sometimes, it's worse. At the end of the day, I can't say for sure whether the image you have of yourself in your head is a positive or a negative distortion until I know how loud your Jim and Bob are relative to each other; however, what I do know and can say with certainty is

that *it is not accurate*! In general, Bob distorts information through his negative filter – noticing only the worse of everything and magnifying the flaws. Jim does exactly the opposite – finding the one thing that seems to support his view that he is all that and a bag of chips and running with it, regardless of reality.

- Convinced yet? I could go on if you like....

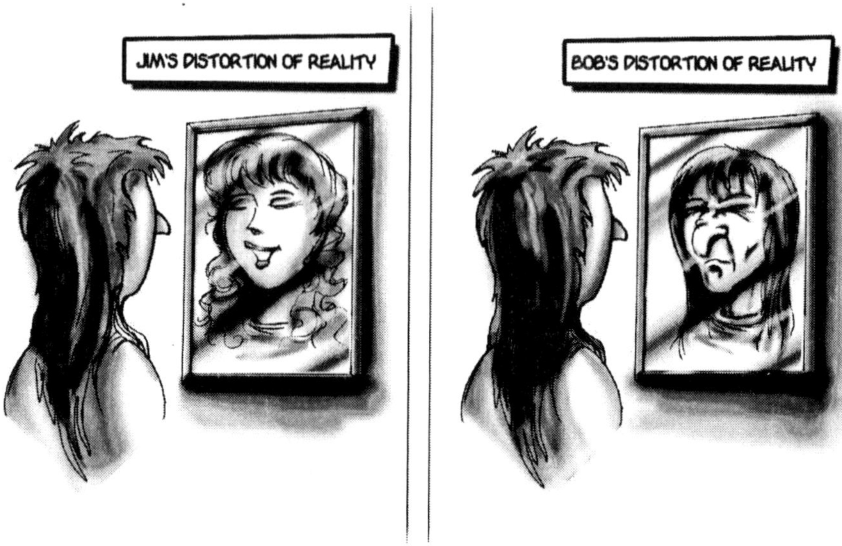

So, at the end of the day, even though you may very well have more information about you than anyone else out there, all of that information is twisted, warped and inaccurate! This essentially makes you *the worst person* in the world to use as a judge of yourself since even though you know a lot about you, none of it is accurate! The fact is that in life, ***we have to rely on others' opinion of us in order to develop an accurate 'Self' image.***

Which bring us to Fact # 3...

Fact #3:

The Majority Rules! a.k.a. The 15% Rule

15% of people in the world will like you and see you in a positive light no matter what you do or what you are like as a person... **AND** ... 15% of people in the world will *NOT* like you and will see you in a ***negative*** light no matter what you do or what you are like as a person. The other 70% of people in the world will see you in a more realistic light and will either like you or dislike you depending on the kind of person that you really are... for really-real!

What this means is that *at best, you will only ever be able to be seen positively by 85% of people* in the world. ***You can't please everyone all the time!!!*** If 85% of people you know say you are attractive, then you are attractive! It does not matter that there is a small handful of people (about 4-5 in a class of 30) who are telling you that you are Fugly. The majority is what is true and real – not the minority! Equally, it does not matter if they happen to agree with what Bob makes you think you think of your 'self' or not – in fact, now you know that *you* are wrong about your 'self' perception... so then, really, who cares if 15 % of people agree with something that is wrong! When listening to others' opinions of us in order to build an accurate self-image, we ***have to rely on the majority opinion!***

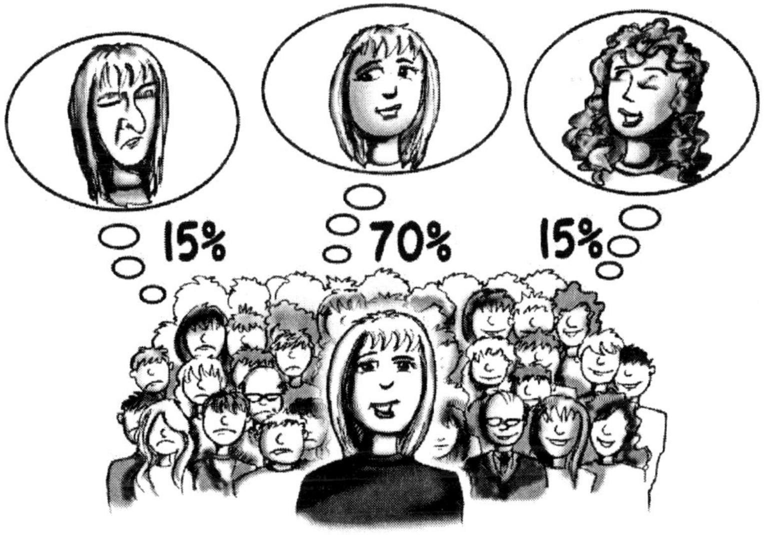

Chapter £Ωα∞€

Are We There Yet?

a.k.a.

The Mental Milestones of Adolescence

Let's Get Mental!

In order to make it through adolescence and become an emotionally well-adjusted adult, there are certain things that need to happen... *you need to win the lottery!* Well, not really... it might help, but it won't make you '*happy*'. What I'm referring to are 7 *things* that you need to figure out... things that you have to learn in order to be able to be successful (emotionally) as you go through puberty and become an adult (*you need to 'get it' in order to get there!*). These things that you need to get don't come all at once. For you to get it, it's going to take time... it takes a good couple of years to *really* get it. For the most part, there is an order to the gettings or at least to starting to get them but this isn't necessarily the order in which they are finished being gotten. (*Have I gotten you confused you yet with getting the gettings and gottens ??? ... or do you get it because you got it?*)

THINGS YOU NEED TO GET TO GET THERE

THE *7 MENTAL MILESTONES OF* ADOLESCENCE

1. ***An accurate mental representation of yourself***

   You need to know who you are... for real (not just who you imagine yourself to be). You need to know... for real... what you can and cannot do based on the body and the brain that you have. Don't forget Rule of the Road #2

2. ***An accurate mental representation of your parents***

   This means that you need to know who/what kinds of people they really are – See Chapters 8, 9 or 10

3. ***An accurate (and forgiving) understanding of human emotions and behaviours***

In other words, being able to understand why you and the other people in your life do the things that you do. It means *understanding "WHY?"* and knowing what it means when you or someone else acts in a certain way. It means understanding what feelings are (just a voice), what they mean (that Bob and Jim are talking loudly – which might not mean *anything!*), and understanding why they are there (because of genetics (out of *your* [Mini-U's] control) and experiences you had in your life, especially those as a child growing up (also out of *your* control)). Then, once you get all of that, applying that knowledge to everything - past, present and future so that you can understand people and the world and life better!

4. **A *'Life Story'***

But not just any story; this story is one that has to make sense to you and has to have a positive 'meaning' or 'moral' at the end for you **AND** your parents. In other words, you need to be able to explain your life to yourself - to find a way to explain/reframe/understand why things in your life happened to you the way they did... **AND** to do this in a way that you can believe/accept **AND** which has a moral/meaning that is **NOT** negative – ***about you or your parents!!!***

5. ***A decision about who/what kind of person you want to be***

This could be as simple as you accepting *who* you are and being OK with it... or it could be as complicated as realizing what kind of person your Harm Avoidance Drive and Pleasure Seeking Drive have already made you and then deciding that you don't want to be that kind of a person and working your butt off to change that into something else... something that *you* decided on. In general, without any intervention from Mini-U, Jim and Bob turn us into our parents... ... ... Scared yet? Not sure if you're scared? Take a good look at your parents; do you like who they are? The kinds of people that they are? The decisions that they make? Do you want to end up being exactly like them? If your answer is "Yes", then that's lucky for you – no work for you to do! If your answer is "#^%@#$* NO!!!", *then start thinking!!!* Start using Mini-U now to change who you are into something else – to *change your "personality"... by changing your behaviour!*

6. ***A realistic plan for your future***

   Realistic means that you have taken into consideration what is real – who you really are, your real strengths and weaknesses, your real supports and challenges, etc.); *to have something that you want to get/achieve in your life* and have it be reasonably possible.

7. ***To find your place in the world***

   In other words, to find acceptance and belonging in a 'group'. For the most part, this is a process that starts in late adolescence (once you have identified who you want to be and where you want to go in life) and often is not successfully completed until your mid-late 20's. This includes that complicated process of finding a partner as well as the process of finding good friends and finding good colleagues.[159]

And that's pretty much it. Get through all that stuff and the rest of your life will be easy. It should be obvious by now that being happy and learning how to be in control of your 'self' is **not** something that will simply happen one day. It is a journey and takes time and effort. But it is, without question, the **most important journey you will ever take!** Have fun getting there and then have fun for the rest of your life too!!!

Take Care of your 'selves' everyone. I hope you got what you were looking for out of this book.

Dr. D

---

[159] people that you work with

Chapter 2.584592

a.k.a

Chapter 13

<u>Is it Platypusses or Platypii?</u>

Hollo! Como es tu? Mucho Gusto?... Si!!! ☺

It's a shame that you are reading this chapter... especially since it would mean that you read the first part all the way through! The truth is, I don't actually expect many people to come to this section... except for those of you who cheat at choose-your-own-adventure books and read ahead before choosing! ... ... you oughta be ashamed of yourselves!

Either way, regardless of why you're here, that's OK because I know that what I tell you in this book is *only* going to be useful to those of you that are willing to *think* about your life, *think* about what you want from life, *think* about who you want to be in life and *decide* to be someone who is in control of their life and in control of their emotions. In other words, those teenagers who are willing to *think and choose the direction of their lives* rather than simply *react to where their lives end up taking them*.

If you are one of those teenagers who has chosen to forfeit using common sense in your life, then I hope that when you eventually get tired of feeling unhappy and angry or sad or worthless or get tired of not being in control of your life and making mistake after mistake after mistake, you decide to pick up this book again and read it all the way through. And I really, really hope that you do this before the age of 22 so that you have a chance to fix your life and make it what you want it to be.

Until then, Via con carne!

Sincerely,

Dr. D.